I0605599

100 Rules for Living to 100

Also by Dick Van Dyke:

Keep Moving

My Lucky Life In and Out of Show Business

100 Rules for Living to 100

AN OPTIMIST'S GUIDE TO A HAPPY LIFE

Dick Van Dyke

WITH TAL McTHENIA

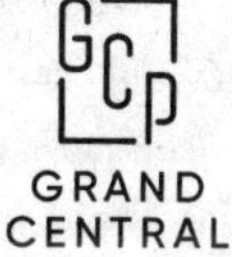

GRAND CENTRAL

NEW YORK BOSTON

Cover design by Dana Li.
Cover photo by Laura Johansen, Alaura Imagery & Design

Photo of Dick with pumpkin by Ray Villafane, Villafane Studios

Grand Central Publishing
Hachette Book Group
1290 Avenue of the Americas
New York, NY 10104
grandcentralpublishing.com
@grandcentralpub

First Edition: November 2025

Grand Central Publishing is a division of Hachette Book Group, Inc. The Grand Central Publishing name and logo are registered trademarks of Hachette Book Group, Inc.

Print book interior design by Timothy Shaner, NightandDayDesign.biz

Library of Congress Cataloging-in-Publication Data has been applied for.

ISBNs: 978-1-538-77790-9 (hardcover); 978-1-538-77792-3 (ebook)

Printed in the United States of America

LSC-C

Printing 3, 2025

To my beautiful wife, Arlene, who edited this book and made my life paradise.

100 Rules for Living to 100

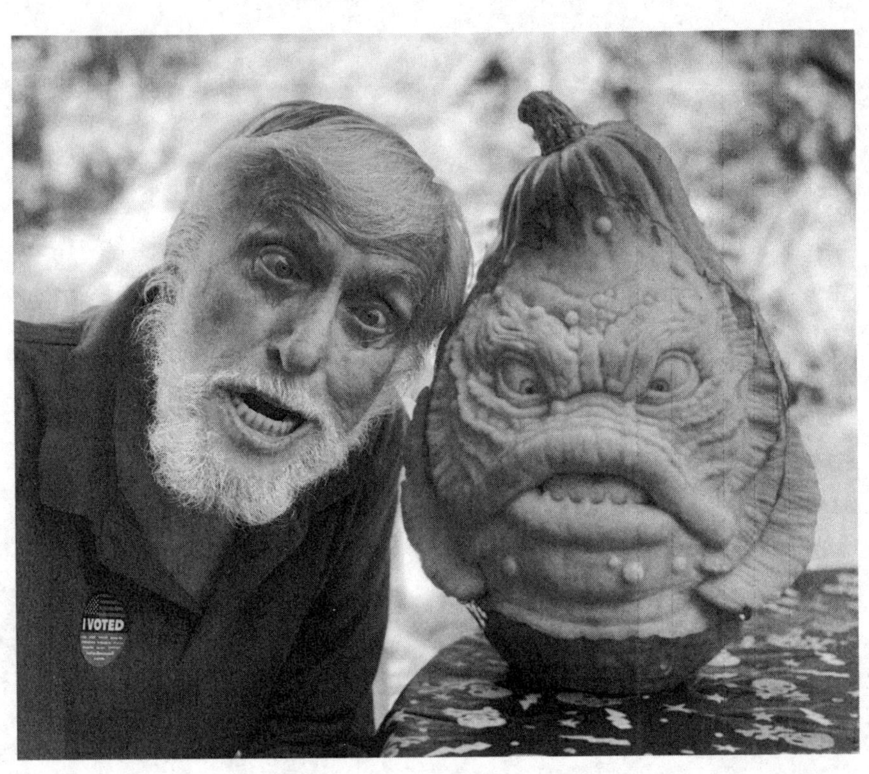
I VOTED

DON'T ACT YOUR AGE

Remember the old man in *Mary Poppins*?

Mr. Dawes Sr. is the greedy, heartless bank president who's the film's only real villain. He's half bald, bearded, hunched over, and wheezy, sporting a shawl around his shoulders to fight a chill and a cane to fight gravity. At the slightest imbalance, he teeters and topples. The man is ancient.

To this day, if you ask who played old Mr. Dawes, an awful lot of people would come up blank. Including those who saw the movie as kids and savvier new generations that are just now discovering it. There's a clue in the credits, where the actor is listed as "Navckid Keyd."

If you're quick with a word scramble, you've guessed correctly that, underneath all that makeup, it was me—not even forty at the time! The role I'm known for in the movie is Bert the Chimney Sweep, so how did I end up with a second part as a senior citizen?

Growing up, I hung around a lot with my grandparents and great-grandparents, and I did a lot of stealth observing. I watched their stoops get stoopier over time, heard their voices get cracklier and thinner. I picked up their old-timey intonations and jargon: "What'd it run ya?" for instance, my great-grandmother's way of asking what something had cost. Thanks to the elders in my family, the "old man" became an early part of my repertoire as a comedian.

So as soon as I read the part of Mr. Dawes, I saw a whole world of comic potential. After begging Walt Disney for the part, even offering to play it for free, he made me do a screen test to confirm that a cheerful, limber thirty-eight-year-old Dick really could transform himself into a sour, stiff nonagenarian. To clinch the deal, I hobbled behind some fake bushes to pee, which broke Walt up.

During breaks from shooting, still in my bald cap and prosthetic makeup, I was unrecognizable to most people on the Disney lot. I pranked tourists on studio tours. Even the two lead child actors had trouble believing that Dawes was actually me.

A few years later, I got a chance to go senior on-screen again in my CBS special, playing Ludwig, the World's Oldest Magician. In this sketch, due to Ludwig's advanced age, every bit in his magic act goes awry or falls flat, which he buttons up with his standard "Sim-sala-bim!" delivered more like: "Oh, whatever!" Ann Morgan Guilbert (who played my neighbor Millie on *The Dick Van Dyke Show*) played Ludwig's assistant, equally long in the tooth and sloppy with her work. Lots of our humor came from how much this old pair, after all these years, thoroughly despised each other.

A decade later, midlife Dick took up geriatric friction again with Carol Burnett on *Van Dyke and Company.* Carol, who was also playing old, ruins an origami duck that it's taken me thirty-seven years to complete. Then—in a spontaneously improvised two-minute addendum to the sketch—we get into a full-on brawl, old-person style, with all our lunging, hitting, falling, and floor-grappling performed in very slow motion.

Now here we are many decades later. I'm ninety-nine; as old if not older than Mr. Dawes, Origami Guy, or Ludwig. I'm not playing a super-old anymore. I *am* a super-old. Speaking now from this position of centenarian authenticity, I can look back on my old man roles and say that some stuff I got right.

Mostly, it's the physical deterioration that feels accurate. Like my old characters, I am now in fact a stooper, a shuffler, and a teeterer. I have feet problems and I go supine as often as is politely possible.

Those fake old-timers smacked their dentures. I chew nicotine gum, all day long—still, decades after I quit smoking!

My sight is so bad now that origami is out of the question. I have trouble following group conversations and complain frequently about my hearing aids, though I would never refer to them as ear trumpets. I'm not *that* old.

At mealtime, I spill stuff, and when my wife Arlene asks me to put on an unstained shirt before we go out, I get impatient.

"It's got blueberry all over it," she'll say.

"Polka dots are in again!" I'll reply.

But the superficial stuff, the physical decay, is about the only thing I share with the old guys I played way back when. Thank God, on the inside, I am as different from them as I could get.

Those guys were just so peppery. And in case that's an old-timey word, let me translate: irritable and sharp-tongued. Get-off-my-lawn kind of guys. The only measly joy they got out of life was through malice against other people. Remember how positively gleeful old Dawes is when his son fires Mr. Banks by punching a fist through his hat?

Also, there was an underlying sadness to a lot of the old guys I played. Their best years were behind them. They were dusty relics, forgotten by the world.

I get all that, I do. Though I still do guest spots on TV, and ads and videos, I miss going to the studio every day for a regular series—work that gave me so much pleasure and purpose. And every single one of my dearest lifelong friends is gone, which feels just as lonely as it sounds.

It's frustrating to feel diminished in the world, physically and socially. I get invites to events or offers for gigs in New York or Chicago, but that kind of travel takes so much out of me that I have to say no. Almost all of my visiting with folks has to happen at my house, and after an hour of conversation, I just crash.

On top of that, recent and unfolding current events could turn anyone sour and dark, young or old. I just lived through two Southern California wildfires in less than a month, right out my front door, including the worst one in history. Daily, I spiral into anguish over the mayhem and cruelty being inflicted on the entire world by those in power.

So yes, I suppose at certain times of day, I am the grumpy old man who yells at the TV.

But that's not the essence of me.

And, frankly, it's not the essence of anybody else, either. No one is a grumpy old man at heart. No one is genetically miserable. No matter our current circumstances, we all have the capacity for a joyful and purposeful life.

If I didn't know that to be true, I wouldn't have written this book.

It's been an intensely eye-opening process, these past many months, reflecting on my ninety-nine years of life, work, and relationships. I've unearthed lost treasures of memory, reconsidered my well-worn stories, connected fragments from my distant past to immediate present, hit upon patterns and themes that span the whole of my life.

But I wasn't doing it just for the sake of navel-gazing. My motivation in remembering and reflecting has been the same as my motivation for performing. Actually, for living overall! To give *other people* something of myself. Specifically, I live with a lifted spirit, and my purpose on earth has been to lift the spirits of my fellow humans.

So, behind all my pondering over the stories in this book, there was always an impatient question: *Yes, Dick, but so what? What good is this to anybody else?!*

I've made it to one hundred, in no small part, because I have stubbornly refused to give in to the bad stuff in life: failures and defeats, personal losses, loneliness and bitterness, the physical and emotional pains of aging. That stuff is real, but I have not let it define me.

Because, as I see it, to do that would be to throw the towel in on life itself.

Instead, for the vast majority of my years, I have been in what I can only describe as a full-on bear hug with the experience of living. Being alive has been *doing life*—not like a job, but rather like a giant playground.

What does my playground look like exactly? What is it about the monkey bars and seesaws that keeps my heart racing? Boiled down, the things that have kept my life joyful and fulfilling are pretty simple: romance, doing what I love, and a whole lot of laughing.

Let me show you what that looks like on the ground, as they say.

To pull the "grumpy old man" away from the TV, my wife Arlene will walk in and dance along to the pharmaceutical ads. This gets me in a musical mood and out of bed, following her to the kitchen. Invariably, one of us will start singing along the way, and the other will join in:

Musical demon, set your honey a-dreamin'.
Won't you play me some rag?

And if it's a good day, which it almost always is in our house, we'll break into a little swaying and soft-shoe right there while she's making lunch.

You'll get all my applause,
And that is simply because I wanna listen to rag.

I met Arlene in 2006, and she quickly became my soulmate and the love of my life. Without question, our ongoing romance is the most important reason I have not withered away into a hermetic grouch.

Arlene is half my age, and she makes me feel somewhere between two-thirds and three-quarters my age, which is still saying a lot. Every day she finds a new way to keep me up and moving, bright and hopeful and needed.

She asks me for a specific definition of *contrapuntal*, with examples. She announces that the Halloween store has finally reopened, and we've got to get over there fast. She gets me to tell stories we both know she's heard a million times before, but how can I resist Arlene?

Arlene is my partner in love, life, and logistics. She has two phones and is often on both, scheduling and juggling more gigs and get-togethers than you could possibly imagine. Arlene knows how much performing and being social nourishes my spirit and brings me alive. I would absolutely be origami guy if she didn't have me singing and dancing.

That little Irving Berlin number we were just singing together in the kitchen? That's one of the tunes we'll be performing next month with my a capella group The Vantastix. Last month, we attempted it during our first gig after a long dry spell, and we were a bit rusty.

By *we*, I mostly mean "me." Yes, for trickier numbers like that, I can miss my cue. Or I'll forget some lyrics. Or come in a little off-key. But none of that gets in my way. If I fall off during a song, I grab on again as soon as I can. If I'm off-key, I feel my way back on. The lyrics I do remember, I belt.

My fellow Vantastix are all decades younger than me, which also has had a rejuvenating effect, these twenty-five years we've been together. When we sing, my heart just soars. Because I'm still doing what I love.

And on to the final ride feature of playground life: laughing. In high school, I schemed elaborately silly pranks with my buddies, and on *The Dick Van Dyke Show*, it was the same feeling—all of us coming up with more and more outlandish ways to make one another lose it.

The guy who used to make me laugh the most, Carl Reiner, is gone now. But I've still got to scratch that itch somehow!

Luckily, I have Jimmy, our assistant, who is forty-one years old, full of secret mischief just like me, and the ideal audience for testing out material. Also, as I get older, I have found that life is more and more a comedy of errors. So if you can't laugh at yourself, you've got big problems.

This brings me back to humorless old Mr. Dawes. There's only one scene where his character comes close to the old man I'm living right now. It's when he hears a joke from earlier in the movie, now retold by Mr. Banks, whom he's just fired.

BERT: I know a man with a wooden leg named Smith.
UNCLE ALBERT: What's the name of his other leg?

It takes old Dawes a ridiculously long time to get the joke, but when he does, he starts wheeze-laughing uncontrollably. In an echo of an earlier scene in the movie, the chortling causes him to float up into the air, above the other horrified bankers.

No matter my mood, no matter my pain, a good little joke will boost my spirits. And the more I laugh, the more I'm lifted—if I'm lucky, maybe, right up into the air!

MAKE YOUR OWN RULES

Before we really get going, I need to make a few things clear about this book:

I don't believe in telling other people what to do. So, you're not going to find "biohacks" or "optimization protocols" or anything like that here. I mean, I go to the gym three mornings a week, but I also appreciate your need to sleep in and get your exercise whenever your body eventually tells you it wants that. I like to go barefoot as much as possible because it keeps me sure-footed and comfortable. This practice is called "earthing" and I highly recommend it, but if shoes are your thing, that's fine by me.

The "rules" in this book aren't about physical stuff, anyway. Nor do they form a step-by-step guide, because that would be ridiculous. If I've learned anything, it's that the world has a sneaky way of upending all our plans, no matter how well laid.

The rules here are about living and being *within* our ever-shifting circumstances. Going with the flow, yes, but also making the most of it. Finding, in the flow, our greatest sense of joy, fulfillment, and purpose.

Each rule springs from a story from my own life, which I believe has stuck itself in my memory for a good reason—because it has some broader emotional significance for me to ponder. For *us* to ponder, together. Not exactly prescriptive "life lessons," but often more like "life questions." Stuff I'm batting around that I think you'd benefit from batting around too. Sometimes I'll try to tell you what I think the rule is about, for me, but it's up to you to make it work for you, however you see fit.

I readily admit that you might find variations of the same rule emerging in multiple stories here. That's because my life, like everyone else's, has its personality-specific ongoing themes—questions that pop up, over and over again, in different contexts, old challenges that look different in each new light, wisdom learned and forgotten and learned again.

I might also add that, for some of these stories, there's not exactly a rule or even a specific question. Sometimes that's because I know there's some nugget of meaning in the story, but I haven't quite figured out what it is. Maybe you can! Other times, it's just a funny story, plain and simple. Because don't we all sometimes just need comic relief?

Finally, if you're inclined to count up these rules to see if there are exactly one hundred, as advertised in the title, your math might disappoint you, just a little. Quality over quantity, as the saying goes, right? I can assure you that this book will deliver enough main rules, sub-rules, ancillary rules, and multipart rules to last you a lifetime, yes, all the way to one hundred!

And anyway, the title of this chapter is "Make Your Own Rules." Which is precisely what I'm doing!

EXAMINE YOUR HEAD

Recently, I got a letter or something about a study into extreme human aging and why some people live for so long. Scientists have discovered that from ninety-nine on, well, there's a lot they don't know. They can't figure out why some people are living so long, especially people who still have some marbles.

I still have marbles, and I'm still mobile, so I'd make an ideal subject. I was going to sign up for the study because I'm sure they would have wanted to use me, but I lost the thing.

Okay, I admit. My short-term memory is shot—names, where I put things, what happened yesterday. But at least I can tell when I'm repeating what I just said ten minutes ago: instead of saying "Wow! What?!" people just say "Mm-hmm." So, I feel like that counts for something in the cognition department, right?

This morning, I got Arlene helping me to remember what this study was and find it online, but she wasn't having any luck. "National Institute on Aging? Extreme heat? No," she read aloud, searching her phone.

"They'd probably put a lot of electrodes on your head anyway," I reasoned, ready to give up.

"Well, you definitely need to be studied," Arlene insisted, still searching.

She'd given me the seeds for a quip. "Oh, so you think I ought to have my head examined, is that what you're saying?"

"No," Arlene laughed. "I mean: studied for why you are the way you are. *Why* are you the way you are?"

Well, probably because I stopped drinking a long time ago, which must have saved a lot of brain cells. I used to do the crossword religiously for years (in pen), and now it's *Jeopardy!* that keeps me sharp, though Arlene always has the answers before I do. Apparently, there are these "superfoods" that are good for brain health, so maybe I've ingested a lot of those?

The biggest reason I can think of is my ability to memorize. For my whole career, I had to memorize pages and pages of lines and a ton of songs, backward and forward, so I was able to say or sing them without even thinking.

When I sing with The Vantastix, it's often songs from shows and movies I've done, and those are right at the front of my brain. I can still pick up new material easily, too, though it might take three or four more run-throughs than it used to before the lyrics feel like second nature. Also, I'm not afraid to forget a word or two, as long as I can keep up the tune.

"Did you find anything yet?" I asked Arlene, still pecking away at her phone.

"What? No, I just got eleven texts."

I rolled my eyes.

So maybe that's my secret, then. For a decade now, the only cell phone in my life has been Arlene's, and she's the one who actually operates it. She gave me this thing called "Alexa," but as soon as I found out Alexa was a spy, she was unplugged and banished. I do have an iPad, but I don't text or shop or browse for hours on end. Think of all the dopamine I've stored up!

LEARN TO FALL

Imagine you're a toddler again. You've been standing up on your hindquarters for some time now, so you're mostly steady. Still, sometimes gravity gets the better of you, and you tip forward a little, and then some more, until you're definitely going over. Your face is just a second away from smashing into the kitchen floor.

Quick! What do you do?!

If you answered, "Put out your hands!" you're like most people in the world. This is a thing called the parachute reflex, and a child typically develops it between five and nine months of age. That's before they can stand even, when they're still crawling and belly-squirming.

As a child, my answer to that question would have been: "Absolutely nothing." According to my mother's firsthand accounts, during my very early years, I would never break my falls. I'd just land on my face or my belly and start crying. Then do it again a few minutes later.

With my mother's guidance, I had to consciously learn this simple technique of self-protection. It wasn't a reflex I could trust. It was a muscle I had to build.

But once I built it, *watch out*! Once I got a little older, knowing how to fall safely, and knowing I knew how to fall safely, opened up a lot of possibilities—for falling *for fun*! What a rush that was! Of course, I wanted to fall all the time!

On Saturday afternoons, my buddies and I spent all day in the movie theater watching cowboy and cops-and-robbers pictures, studying all the ways a shot-up crook or gunslinger could collapse and die. Then we ran home to try out the moves ourselves in the backyard. I learned then that I had a knack for more than just simple falling, but the elaborate pre-fall stagger, too; the collapse-to-the-knee fall; giving every fall a special little twist, replete with winces, groans, and wound-clutching.

When it came to putting the *comedy* into falling, that's something I learned from Buster Keaton, whose classic old shorts and silents were a must-see whenever the theater ran them. His pratfalls were in a category all their own. He had this hysterical way of throwing his legs up in the air when he fell on his back. And he took the most epic head-over-heels tumbles.

Much later in life, I got the secrets to these tricks straight from the master's mouth. Buster was in his sixties at the time, living out in the Valley. I was so eager to meet him that I called him up cold—and he invited me over for a cookout!

In his big backyard, Buster grilled hot dogs and delivered them by toy train to the table—I adored him immediately. Eventually, the conversation got around to pratfalls, successful and not. He told me that at one time or another, he had broken every bone in his body, including his neck. It turns out his legs in the air bit was to throw all the weight onto his shoulders, as opposed to his back. And as for falling forward, here was his big secret: You don't just hit the ground flat, you sort of tuck in and roll into the fall.

By that time, I was doing my own slips and flops and topples on *The Dick Van Dyke Show*, and Buster's advice came in handy. In our first season, Carl Reiner came to appreciate my gift, and we worked clumsiness into my character. In one episode alone, I tripped and fell over a toy fire truck, my briefcase, and a card table.

This led to the fall that would become my most well-known: the trip over the ottoman in the show's opening credit sequence.

In season one, the credits had rolled over still photos of the cast in action, which Carl got bored with. For our next season, he wanted something funnier, with a spark. So, in a kind of spur-of-the-moment thing, he gathered up the cast and crew and director John Rich in the main living room set to shoot a new opening.

To this day, I'm not sure who came up with the idea, me, Carl, or somebody else. Like the best ideas on that show, it felt like it came from all of us. Rob would come home from work where Laura (his wife) and Buddy and Sally (his comedy writer pals) were waiting, step over to greet them, and promptly trip over the ottoman.

I did it in one take! I wasn't using Buster's training, either.

John called cut and print, but rather urgently. Unbeknownst to any of us, he had a date that night out in Malibu and was itching to get out of there.

But then Carl had another idea, and John sighed. He wanted a variation on the opening where I almost trip, then swerve around the ottoman instead. Then, we would switch up the two openings, week to week, so the audience would never know which one they'd get.

We filmed that second one, too, in one take. So, after all of four or five minutes, John was off to his date.

As real fans of the show might know, there's a third variation on the opening that appears only rarely, where I avoid the ottoman but then end up tripping and stumbling anyway. Of course.

That little trick of Carl's got so popular that each week, people would bet, with actual money, on whether I would fall or not.

Over the years, I've fallen more ways than I can count. I wish someone would do one of those compilation videos of every single one of them ever captured on camera. It would go on for hours.

I'm ninety-nine now, and people are still asking me if I can fall like I used to. Ha. Ha.

"I sure can," I reply, "but it hurts more now."

FIND YOUR PASSION IN YOUR PAST

At this advanced age, my very sharpest life memories are of childhood. I am sure there are hard neuroscientific reasons for this phenomenon, but I think maybe something more mysterious is going on too.

Recently, out of nowhere, I got a few flashes from my early youth that felt "fresh." A memory not in my familiar repertoire. So, I kept my mind there, and let the flashes unspool:

My little hands, slathering gray paint onto a cut-out cardboard tombstone. Then another and another. Painting a cardboard triangle-topped building—a house? a church?

Putting on some kind of dark cloak. Holding a big shovel. Slinking among the cardboard graves, getting spooked by something and shrieking—very over-the-top.

My third- or fourth-grade classmates cracking up. Their reactions emboldening me to keep getting hammier. Wielding my shovel like a weapon at whatever was threatening me.

More laughter, much louder.

Don't ask me the plot of this little grade school play, don't ask about other characters—trust me, I've tried to rustle those details up already.

Why does this school play stand out so distinctly? Not just because it was an unusual occasion, it's got to be more than that. After some leisurely pondering, it hit me:

This is my very first memory of doing something I love.

Really, really love.

Building sets, creating costumes, contorting my body, face and voice for comedy, feeding off my audience. This was my first true passion.

And all these years, my brain has been holding on to that memory, protecting it, so I could connect with it and reap its power.

For most of my life, that's been a passive, indirect process. While this specific memory must have popped up at earlier times in my life (that I now can't recall), I don't think I consciously appreciated its whole meaning until now. Still, it must have always been back there, bubbling its way into my instincts and life choices.

How else can I explain the following:

In high school, I considered a future in sports. I trained to become an Air Force pilot. I worked in advertising. I had looong spells of doubt during my early entertainment career. Later in life, I contemplated retiring out to sea on my sailboat. Even just fifteen years ago, before I met Arlene, I thought maybe I should just pack showbiz up and fritter away at home.

Yet, at each and every one of these points in my life, something rose up inside me, shook me and admonished me: *No, Dick. This is not what you love. This is not who you are.* Like I was about to build my house out in the yard, not on its foundation.

In these moments, I could sense I was veering off track because I knew what being *on track* felt like. I knew what it was I *did* love to do.

It occurs to me that since the memory of doing that little graveyard act was always there inside me, I could have tapped into it more actively and consciously had I appreciated just how powerful and significant it was.

I have "worked with" my childhood memories before in life, but usually it's the bad stuff. In my forties, I went into treatment for my alcoholism (which you'll hear about later), and as part of therapy, I pulled up buried memories of some really painful family times when I was young. This excavation was a big help in unpacking and working through my adult emotional struggles.

But why should I, or anyone, limit this exercise to working through pain? Can't we also use our memories to connect or reconnect ourselves to our passions? What I'm saying now—to you—is that you've got a chance to be proactive about this whole thing in a way I wasn't.

Before I explain, a warning: There's an emotional risk involved here, and if you're in a delicate place, this activity is not recommended. Stop reading now. Even if you think you're fine, proceed with caution and know that I'll talk you through it on the other side.

Here we go.

Relax your mind. Take your thoughts back to childhood. And ask yourself, specifically: *What is my first memory of doing something I love?*

To be clear, I'm not talking about just your "happiest" memories, e.g., Christmas morning. Look for times when you're *doing the thing* that makes you the happiest.

Call up as many little flashes of this activity as you can—those are clues! Remember the doing, but also the feeling! Don't worry too much about turning the memory into a narrative; there's time for that later. Right now, just gather the clues. You can spread this out over days, weeks, months, even years! However you do it, *hold on* to what you remember (a thing I have to tell myself all the time).

Once you've had time to really process the memory, you're ready for the harder part: comparing it to your present.

If the key elements of that childhood pursuit match up with, or clearly relate to what you're doing now, I'd say you're in good shape. Chances are you're at least in the ballpark of happy.

If they don't match up at all, I realize that is a very weighty and painful thing to discover. Remember, you don't have to do anything big about it, or anything at all; and it will help to talk about it with someone you love.

If you're in a time of active doubt, a life transition, or a moment of big decision-making, this memory can give you a clue about how to proceed. To seek out a future that's closer to doing what you now know you love most purely.

But look. I'm not suggesting you have to rethink and upend your entire life! "I used to love climbing trees! Goodbye job, goodbye family! Annapurna here I come!"

There are simpler options, at your fingertips. You can use that memory to guide you back to beloved old hobbies, to take a cooking class, go out dancing more on the weekends, spend an hour at a rock-climbing gym.

However and whenever you decide to make use of that memory, it will be there for you. Think of it as your beacon.

Now, if you'll excuse me, I have a new monster to make for Halloween.

TOLERATE AND CHERISH YOUR LITTLE BROTHER

From the moment my only other sibling was born, almost six years after me, I was his protector. Some of this was my own doing: Jerry was adorably vulnerable, and it was so satisfying to soothe him with cuddles and cradle-rocking.

Some of this was also a job: early in his life, my parents appointed me his babysitter/nanny—watching him when they were out, putting him to bed, waking him up and getting him dressed. I took the role very seriously too. Alone at night while Jerry slept, I stayed wide-eyed awake, guarding him from the groaning ghosts that filled our empty house, an axe in my grip.

Later, the sibling dynamic got more complicated. Starting when I was still in the single digits, most of the heavy manual labor in our house fell on me. My traveling salesman father was gone six days a week, my mother had her hands full running the rest of the household, and Jerry was still too young to be anything but an enthusiastic chore-watcher or chore-beneficiary. Which sometimes rubbed me the wrong way.

Case in point, my most wretched chore of all, which in Jerry's mind was "The Big Brother Coal Show!" Winters in

Danville, Illinois, were long and vicious, and nearly all the houses in town were heated by coal furnaces. Back then, we used soft coal—the messy kind.

While Jerry was blissfully dreaming away at night, I was down in the basement shoveling load after load of those filthy black chunks into the furnace, then tamping the furnace down to smolder all night. In the morning when the house was arctic, Jerry was lingering under his toasty covers while I was back in the basement, getting the furnace going. As the heat made its way up into the house, my mother and I would rush to one of the floor vents and stand there shivering, waiting for the first warmth to hit our toes and legs, before darting off to our other morning duties. Meanwhile, Jerry was free to stroll downstairs and take his spot on a vent only after the heat was really blasting.

By midwinter, it was time for Jerry's favorite part of my coal show: cleaning the furnace and taking the ashes out, along with the hardened nuggets of coal by-product known as "clinkers." For this, Jerry had a front-row seat on the basement steps, delighting in his brother's unhappy mess—clothes, hands and arms and face, smeared with black soot.

And, in springtime was the finale! Out came the rags and a jar of the "pink stuff": a pink paste cleaner that Jerry found totally fascinating. Watching me scrub it across our soot-covered walls—every single wall, plastered or wallpapered, every room in the house, floor to ceiling, yes, the ceiling!—he marveled at the magical transformation.

Looking up at me, perched on the very top rung of a ladder and nursing an arm cramp, Jerry would helpfully point out that three-quarters of the ceiling soot had yet to vanish. "Why'd you stop?"

In the summer, there was still work for me to do and Jerry to watch, but there were other things we got to share as equals. Endless afternoons of carefree play with the other kids in the street or someone's backyard. With that came another essential and cherished brotherly ritual: ice, coal's cleaner summer counterpart.

Danville summers were scorching and humid, and back then, there was no air-conditioning. So, while the primary purpose of ice was to refrigerate our food, that was kind of an abstraction to us kids. Jerry and I loved ice for all its more tangible palliative powers.

It arrived almost daily to our house via horse-drawn wagon, piled high with big ice blocks of various weights. Most everybody ordered twenty-five-pound cubes for their ice boxes, which meant the iceman was always chipping them off from the bigger blocks.

Invariably, stray chunks or shards would break off and pile up in the back of the truck. So, while the ice man was delivering a cube into the house to the icebox, Jerry and I would climb up in the back of the truck and snatch up as many scraps as we could before the driver came back.

The small chunks were good for rubbing on our sunburned arms and necks and slipping down each other's shirts. The bigger shards were the perfect thirst-quencher. We could slurp on those things forever.

One afternoon, I heard the ice man returning from our house and scampered off the wagon, but Jerry was too lost in his ice revelry to follow. Oblivious to his little stowaway, the ice man hopped in front and got the horses going. Panicked, I sprinted after them, but before I could get the driver's attention, my brother toppled out of the wagon and onto the street with a horrifying *thwonk* to his head.

When I reached Jerry lying there, he was fully conscious, thank God, on his way from stunned silence to loud hysteria. His bawling reached my mother, who ran out, scooped him up and carried him inside. Miraculously, after a visit from the doctor and a day of careful monitoring, Jerry turned out to be fine, save some scrapes and a lump on his head, which meant—for him—a consolation prize of more ice from our box.

After that, the back of the ice truck was off-limits, but the iceman—likely feeling guilty—always kept me and Jerry well-stocked with scraps.

I felt guilty too. I'd failed Jerry in my most important role: his protector. For years after his fall, well into my adolescence, it would nag at me. I would catch myself studying how Jerry moved and talked, searching with dread for any signs of brain damage that the doctor had missed.

A few winters after the accident, Jerry was becoming more of a chore-*doer* himself, and he wanted to climb the ladder and play with the pink stuff. Sure, part of me was relieved that my little brother might soon be able to take over some of my work. But part of me wanted him to just stay down on the floor like he always had, watching safely.

"Next year," I told him. "When you're older."

This complex brotherly dynamic persisted for our entire lives. Sometimes Jerry was the "chore-beneficiary," sometimes I was the "protector," and sometimes we just played together as equals.

After I'd broken into live comedy, Jerry (who was pretty aimless at the time) saw my act and decided that's what he wanted to do, too, then promptly stole all my material! After my first television appearance in LA, I wrote Jerry, urging him to get into TV himself. On *The Dick Van Dyke Show*, I talked Jerry's comedy chops up to the show's creator Carl Reiner, who brought him on board to guest star as my TV brother.

Whenever Jerry and I worked together, we brought our real-life brotherly dynamics into our performances and it was a hoot. In 2011, he cajoled me into costarring with him in a production of Neil Simon's comedy *The Sunshine Boys* at the Malibu Playhouse (our first time doing theater together). We played an estranged old vaudeville duo, trying for a reunion comeback on TV. Jerry was seventy-nine, I was eighty-five, and for the whole show, pretty much, all we did was cleverly bicker. Once, we were running our lines backstage and Arlene's mother, whom she had brought by for a visit, thought Jerry and I were fighting for real! Night after night, we ripped each other apart like we never would dream of doing in real life, and it was so cathartic.

Since Jerry and his wife Shirley weren't living in Los Angeles at the time, Arlene and I invited them to stay in our guest house for rehearsals and the run of the show. Then, Jerry's role on ABC's *The Middle* turned into a recurring one and he wrote in a part for me, so their visit became an extended residency. This was the longest we'd spent together in our entire adult lives, and honestly, at first, I was at a loss for how to even talk to my brother. But we found a comfortable rapport and rhythm, and in retrospect, that never-ending sleepover with my little brother is something I truly cherish.

When Jerry died in 2018, I grieved the loss of our eternally paradoxical relationship. True to form, much of this grieving took the form of laughter—morbid laughter, Jerry's favorite. You may have heard me tell this story before, but in this context, it's too good to resist a repeat.

Back in the early 2000s, when Jerry was on the waitlist for a new kidney, I had arranged to donate mine to him if I died. Every morning, I would answer the phone and it was Jerry, disappointed.

"Oh, you're still alive."

FACE YOUR FEAR

One Saturday afternoon when I was eleven or twelve, I was scrounging around the sidewalks of downtown Danville for movie money. I needed fifteen cents to get into a matinee, but three blocks into my search, I'd come up empty. Then, just outside the drugstore, a silver glint caught my eye. A whole quarter! Now I had popcorn money too!

I snatched it up and raced down the street, right into the theater, not even looking up at the marquee. It never mattered what was playing, anyway; if I had the money, I'd see it. Hopefully, today I'd get a Western.

Popcorn in hand, I settled into my seat just as the movie was starting—with a smirking bow-tied man addressing the camera: "Mr. Carl Laemmle feels it would be a little unkind to present this picture without just a word of friendly warning."

I shifted in my seat. This wasn't a Western.

"We are about to unfold the story of Frankenstein," the man went on, "a man of science who sought to create a man after his own image without reckoning upon God."

Frankenstein. What had I gotten myself into? The movie had been first released in 1931 (though I didn't know that at the time) and over those six years, only the vaguest impressions of it had filtered down to me. Namely, that it was scary.

"I think it will thrill you. It may shock you. It might even horrify you. So, if any of you feel that you do not care to subject your nerves to such a strain, now is your chance to—" He chuckled mischievously before continuing: "Well, we've warned you."

I stood up from my seat, ready to heed the man's warning and make a run for it. I was already terrified of those noisy ghosts in our house. I didn't need another childhood fear, I really, really didn't.

And yet, my feet couldn't move. My eyes were riveted to the screen.

The movie began with the eponymous "man of science" and his cruel sidekick digging up graves, harvesting body parts and stealing a brain in a jar, and it only got worse from there. When Boris Karloff made his first appearance as Dr. Frankenstein's newly alive experiment—the unibrow, the whites of his eyes, the gruesome stitching scars and the bolts in his neck—you wouldn't believe the shrieks that filled that little movie house. Other children skittered out, and even some adults.

Still standing at my seat, I registered this exodus and felt a little tingle of revelation. I wasn't running out. Not that I wasn't petrified. But maybe I was also brave.

Karloff's lurching, thumping gait, his ghoulish fingers, the sheer size of him: here was a monster unlike anything we'd ever seen before, and he seared himself deep into my young psyche. Just as bad were the noises he made, his grunts and moans, his raging roars and high howls of agony.

I never sat down, but I never looked away.

When the movie was finally over, I wobbled out of the theater, and it was already dark. I had a two-mile walk home, alone. My heart sank.

Out here, in the real world, the movie monster couldn't get me. But some other ghoulish creature or phantom certainly could, or even a human killer. Now I wasn't just scared of house ghosts and Boris Karloff, I was scared of everything! Things I couldn't even see!

That long dark walk was agony. I kept myself right in the middle of the street, on high alert, giving myself as wide a berth as possible from whatever might be lurking behind those trees and in those bushes. I tried to recall my bravery from the movie theater, but every little noise or movement gave me a start.

At home in bed that night, I hid myself under the covers and shut my eyes against the terror, but when I finally fell asleep, they all came back again in nightmares. Night after night, for weeks.

Eventually, I was able to let it sink in that my nightmares were not real—an obvious thing that I thought I'd learned years ago! And, in the daytime, I retraced my long walk home, studying the trees and bushes, forcing myself to see how harmless they really were, cementing that knowledge through repetition.

I was learning something about myself. Not just that I was brave. But I was resilient. I was careful. Fear was something I could control.

I'm not recommending that parents trot their kids out to horror movies to teach them the value of fear. To this day, I wonder what that theater manager was thinking, showing such a thing for a Saturday matinee to a theater full of kids!

But when childhood fears do arise, they shouldn't be hidden from and bottled up. They should be faced, talked through, and deconstructed. I wish I'd had more help from my parents in that department, but I suppose going it alone was part of my lesson too.

As you'll soon read, my childhood exploration of fear later blossomed into an obsession with Halloween, specifically the scarier parts of the holiday. Remember that monster I was planning two chapters ago? That's me, every October, finding new ways to push the fear button—in other people and in myself. For my whole life, I've been putting myself back in that movie theater, standing there frozen, feeling out the difference between "too terrified to sit" and "too excited to run."

More immediately, in my early adolescence, I got something else from working through my fears: a little insight into the human condition. Once my young mind had successfully separated fantasy from reality, I was now able to tap into, and explore, a much deeper unease I'd been holding on to about *Frankenstein*.

Specifically, Boris Karloff's nuanced, tragic portrayal of the monster, which I relived over and over in bed at night, now that I was no longer hiding under my pillow. I realized, in fact, that he wasn't a monster at all! He was a human. Misjudged by his appearance and misunderstood. He went rogue and crazy and bad because of the way people treated him. And if they had just tried to understand him, to be decent . . . well, maybe he could have ended up a nice guy.

I began to let this insight filter out into some bigger picture thinking. At its heart, fear—and all the other horrible things that can follow it—is based on not knowing. That's something I would be chewing on for the rest of my life.

FIND "THE NEW YOU" INSIDE "THE OLD YOU"

A lot of comedians got their start doing magic—Johnny Carson, Steve Martin, Jason Alexander, and yours truly. Some people say it's because magic tricks and jokes are kind of the same structure—setup, build, punch line or poof! Once you have that rhythm in your bones as a performer, it's a natural crossover.

For me, the switch from illusions to laughs happened totally by accident. And it involved something harder to describe than a simple familiarity of form. It was the result of all kinds of young emotional and creative growth happening inside me, with my conscious mind playing catch-up. Almost a century later, I think I can finally trace that line.

My love of trickery started when I was a little kid and saw a magic show for the first time. Some folks can just enjoy the illusion and leave it at that. But I was in the category of kid who needed to figure out how it was done.

At first, I just experimented on my own—hiding things in my sleeve, building a secret panel inside an old top hat—but I didn't get far without an instruction book. Luckily, my mother picked up on my new interest, and for Christmas that year, I got a whole magic set. I practiced all the tricks for hours in front of the mirror. Pretty soon, I got really good at palming things—coins, handkerchiefs, cards. There was a bowl-and-water trick I loved too.

For many Christmases after that, I got a new magic set with a fresh set of tricks to master. This was the Depression, so the magic kit was the only present I got. Which was fine by me.

When I was around twelve, I took my act public, setting up my little table of tricks at the ladies lunches held at our local Kiwanis club (a charitable service organization). I pulled in three dollars a show! Being mothers themselves, the ladies were an adoring and forgiving audience; they dutifully gasped and tittered as coins vanished behind my handkerchief and reappeared behind their ears.

But looking back it felt like maybe there was another layer to their delight with me. They seemed surprised that a twelve-year-old boy could be so warm and well-spoken. I was connecting with them not as mothers, but as people, maybe even peers. As a performer, I realize I was learning the power of charm.

After that, I discovered another key element of the magician's persona: "cool." Oddly enough, there was a club of hobbyist magicians in Danville, adult men—local store owners and businessmen—and they got wind of my talent (from their wives, I guess) and invited me to join them. I was all of thirteen at the time, the only kid in the club, and right away they made me their project. Their technical tips were amazing (many, beyond my abilities), and they showed me how to keep my pre-trick patter feeling fresh.

But their lessons in demeanor were most important. As successfully as I had charmed the Kiwanis ladies, the men spotted in my act tiny hints of struggle—a card fumble here, a stammer there—that would, if unchecked, accumulate into a fatal failure of audience trust. Meaning, they wouldn't "buy" my illusions. If I couldn't stop myself from sweating, my Magic Elders declared, I needed to get better at hiding it.

So it was then that I began to cultivate an air of composure. At home and at magic club practices, I worked to make every little wrist movement graceful, every word assured, until the Elders were finally impressed.

Not long after this suave persona was born, though, it was thoroughly dismantled.

At around fifteen, I landed my biggest venue yet for performing my magic: the high school assembly, an audience of 1,400 students. At Danville High, assembly was a showcase for the performing arts, whether it was a traveling orchestra or a drama club skit. It was a cherished part of our school culture, and everyone took their performances very seriously.

For my assembly act, I decided on an illusion I'd recently mastered and felt sure would wow: the Egg Bag Trick, which involved making an egg disappear in a "magic bag." At home to prepare, I hollowed out two raw eggs by poking holes in either end, then blowing out the yolks. I practiced the trick and my patter, turned on the charm and kept my cool.

As I strode onstage—my smile easy and assured—I was pretty sure I was making the right first impression. I set the bag and two eggs on a table, then launched into my intro, feeling each syllable as I hit it.

Then, in my peripheral vision, I detected some unexpected movement. But I knew that faltering equaled death, so I kept my gaze ahead and continued talking. Then my brain processed what I'd just glimpsed—my two eggs slowly rolling across the table—and even then, I didn't break composure.

Only when I heard a nervous titter from the audience, followed by a pair of sad little crunches on the stage floor, did I give in to the reality of failure. I followed my audience's eyes over to my eggs, cracked, misshapen, and saggy. I felt total shame.

With that, the giggles turned into guffaws and hoots, roaring through the auditorium. I turned back to face the crowd and in that split second—though I didn't consciously know it at the time—I made a pretty big discovery about myself.

Yes, cool and charming can be a winning bit. But maybe it's only the setup! When that carefully constructed persona cracks and falls apart, it's funny as hell . . . and maybe that's what my "magic act" really is.

On instinct, I let this new persona spread its wings. Others might have skulked into the wings, humiliated. Instead, I took a deep bow, then walked triumphantly off the stage, as if nothing had gone wrong at all.

The crowd went wild. This time, I *really* had them.

All these years later, now that I see my bridge from magic to comedy, it's as bright as the Vegas Strip. In trying at magic, I found my tools and ingredients as a performer. In failing at magic, I landed the role of a lifetime. I mean, what is Rob Petrie's ottoman trip, if not the perfection of the high school egg fail?

FIND YOUR PEOPLE—A STORY IN SEVERAL PARTS

At certain lucky moments in my life, I have stumbled into a group of strangers that felt like kindred spirits. We developed weird languages together. Our parts formed a mysteriously much greater whole. I adored these other souls ferociously, because I'd never felt so happy or known before in my life.

I've always thought of this experience as "finding my people." Hopefully, it's happened to you too.

Then, just as randomly as I have found them, I have let them slip through my fingers. Not because of some dramatic rupture, but because life just changes and we go our separate ways. Has this part happened to you too? It hurts, doesn't it?

Eventually, we might find more magical clusters like this later in life. Or we might spend the rest of our lives kicking ourselves for losing that first group. Or worse, convincing ourselves that this deep kinship we pine for is just a nostalgic delusion. A connection that couldn't have possibly been that perfect; something we must have dreamed.

Nonsense, I say! In all of the kindred collectives I've been part of, the bonds were real and life-changing. And, if not perfect, then perfect enough in the moment.

That last bit—"perfect enough in the moment" is important. It's the moments we shared together, sometimes very fleeting moments, that stand out most in my memory. And in pondering what those tiny slivers of collective experience are all about, I think maybe I'm hitting on a breakthrough! A way not to drown in sorrow over the "brothers and sisters" we have let fall away, but to stumble on new ones. *Lots and lots of new ones.*

In high school in Danville, I was not a loner by any stretch of the imagination. I had my theater crowd and my track teammates, and I was perfectly happy. I didn't know I'd been missing anything until I found it.

I can't exactly remember how I met Harold Brown, Bob Hackman, Bob Walker, and Jerry C. Wright, but we hit it off right away. Every time we saw one another, in the halls or at some party, we cracked ourselves up. Risqué twists on stale old jokes. Working wry, high school–specific commentary into the lyrics of popular songs. One-upping one another's physical comedy gags, day after day.

Humor was our way of getting to know one another and ourselves. It felt like a muscle we shared but hadn't known existed. In our early days, of course there was boyish competition, but after that, all our best fun was a fully joint production.

We decided our group needed a name, so we picked "Burford" after a local furniture store. One guy was Uncle Burford, one guy was Grandfather Burford, you get the idea. I don't know why we settled on that name, but I think it was because we thought it sounded funny. Say it to yourself in the mirror—"Burrrfurrrd"—and I dare you not to smile. Okay, maybe I'm biased.

Once we'd found our own language of inside jokes, we branched out to inflict our special brand of humor on the rest of the world. We were constantly getting in trouble, though it wasn't exactly real trouble, more just like dorky mischief.

Out on the streets, we would linger in wait near a bus stop, watch the bus roll in, pick up its passengers, then pull away. At which point we'd dash after it down the sidewalk, waving our arms madly, as if we'd missed the bus and were flagging it to stop. Invariably, a passenger would spot us running alongside and call to the driver, who would pull to a stop to pick up us young stragglers.

Instead, we'd just keep running right past the bus, with our arms still flailing.

I found this prank so enduringly amusing that decades later, on the Disney lot during the filming of *Mary Poppins*, I repeated it in my full old banker getup to buses full of tourists.

At school, too, the Burfords were always on the lookout for little ways to subvert the established order, just for kicks. And one day, purely by chance, we hit upon a doozy. Danville High had marble floors, and we discovered that if we sang together and hit a certain note, we could literally make the building vibrate! So much so that we could feel it! I'm not kidding.

When you realize you have a secret power, how can you resist wielding it? Whenever you possibly can?!

At first, our classmates and teachers thought we were singing so loudly and weirdly just to be silly. But then, they felt the vibration too. And we watched them feel it. The twitches in their step, the wince here and there, heads jerking in confusion, maybe—if we really got going—a wave of shared panic!

Once our secret was out, it lost much of its power. Yet, it was too hard to resist, and we kept at it, day after day, still amusing ourselves wildly, but now earning glowering admonishments from our elders and bored eye rolls from our peers. Eventually, we accepted that our public had turned against us, and we retired the vibration superpower for good.

There's no mystery to how the Burfords broke up: after high school, we all went our separate ways, and our lives filled up with careers, families, and new friends. We did keep in touch, many of us for life, and always rejoiced in our brief but momentous history, the details of which only we remembered or cared about.

Still, I felt the loss. For the next few decades, I had plenty of remarkable collaborations (which you'll hear about later!), but only glimpses of that wondrous, innocent Burford synergy.

Then, in 1960, I lucked into finding another group of Burford-esque playmates, and they knocked my socks off. The experience of collective merriment that was *The Dick Van Dyke Show* feels too big to summarize. I'll ease in by describing a moment in one of our early episodes—which was directly inspired by, and a mirror of, our own brand-new, behind-the-scenes creative fusion.

My character, the comedy writer Rob, comes to work miffed that his wife Laura has been opening his mail at home. Rob's cowriter Buddy immediately sees the comic potential of the situation and suggests they write it as a sketch for the show.

"I know where we can go with this," their colleague Sally says.

And then it's off to the races.

In seconds, the three are acting out the parts for the sketch for the others, finishing one another's sentences, building and riffing, revising and adding bits, upping the ante on the humor, and the scale of the humor, at a breakneck pace.

You can see these three feeling the vibration together! And this is exactly what it was like to work on *The Dick Van Dyke Show* itself, every single day.

"You know, my brother, Jerry, was a terrible sleepwalker," I revealed one day to the cast and writers, regaling them with childhood memories of my brother zombie-walking all the way across town. I could see creator Carl Reiner's wheels turning, then everybody else's wheels turning, and they're peppering me for details, and next thing you know, Rob's sleepwalking brother is a two-part story in the show! Played by my actual sleepwalking brother Jerry, no less!

So many episodes emerged like that, bones that Carl or someone else brought in from real life for all of us to gnaw on together. Marauding woodpecker! Gun in the music box! The more we gnawed, the funnier things got.

Each season swept us all up in this joyful spirit of seat-of-the-pants improvisation, always eager to pull new players into our game. "Let's just veer right into a dance number! Who knows any choreographers?!" "What about a whole Western episode?" "Round up some old radio stars!" "We've got another bit for you, Frank—a dejected bohemian!" Whenever our producer Sheldon Leonard showed up on set to observe our wild comedy-making, he'd sigh with bemusement: "Ah, the otters at play."

We knew the show would come to an end after five seasons—that had been Carl's plan all along. But when it happened, the collective grief was indescribable. We were like atoms, sheared off from our molecule. Carl and I chased that magic with more TV collaborations, and Mary Tyler Moore found it with her own show. Many of us stayed close friends, but there was always—and I mean always—a giant ottoman-shaped hole in our shared heart.

In my later years, I have accumulated a new joyful hive, in the form of my singing group, The Vantastix. We are three middle-aged guys with good voices and one old guy with a decent voice, and we've been performing barbershop and our own a cappella arrangements of classics all for twenty-five years. Later in the book, I'll tell you our accidental "origin story," but right now, what matters is only a single moment.

The magic of singing without accompaniment is when four voices, doing four very different things all on their own, come together to harmonize, and you can feel it through your whole body. A single sound so much bigger and better than the individual parts.

But that's also what's so scary about it. Without a piano, you feel naked, and when the harmonies don't quite work, everybody can hear it. For me, at ninety-nine, it's kind of a fifty-fifty crapshoot. No matter how well prepared I think I am, I might just go wildly off-key when we harmonize.

So when The Vantastix recently gathered for a sound check for an afternoon gig at Dreamland, a local Malibu club, I was already a bit jittery. On top of that, it had been six months since our last show, and we'd only had one scattered rehearsal the day before.

The club was empty, save the staff getting the place open and a photography crew setting up for a shoot. They weren't much of an audience, but their presence did raise the stakes, and as we launched into "Supercalifragilisticexpialidocious," I felt that familiar prickle of performance anxiety.

That jaunty barbershop sound is something you don't hear much these days, so some heads started to turn. The other guys were just bopping through it, and most of the right words were coming out of my mouth, so phew. Even though it was just a rehearsal, we all did our synchronized hopping choreography in our seats (which we used to do standing, when my balance was better).

Finally, we got to the scary part—coming together to harmonize—my heart quickening with each rise in pitch.

Um-diddle-diddle-um-diddleye
Um-diddle-diddle-um-diddleye

My eyes were locked on our bass singer Mike's, practically begging him to carry me through on-key. But no matter how much trust and support we'd all built up over the years, the only thing we could rely on in that moment was our will and ability to make our voices connect.

Um-diddle-diddle-um-diddleye
Um-diddle-diddle-um-diddleye

Connect we did! We harmonized perfectly. We achieved synergy!

We all felt it together and broke out into giddy smiles. For me, it was the Burfords-otters feeling, all over again. And our little audience had felt it too.

That whole place was vibrating.

For weeks, I have been thinking about that moment. I feel like it's trying to tell me something.

Our voices didn't harmonize because of our twenty-five years of togetherness. They harmonized because, in those few seconds, we were able to share the language of a cappella.

And that's what matters most. Even if God forbid, The Vantastix ever fall apart, we each still have that tool for coming together with other singers, in other moments. Put another way, as long as we know *how* to play, we can play with anybody, anytime. For a lifetime or just an afternoon.

So really, why pine for a redo of long-lost perfect togetherness?! Instead, embrace the togetherness we can still have, now. *Right. Now.*

At our local supermarket with Arlene, I linger over a box of Honey Nut Cheerios and channel Carmen McRae: "When a bee lies sleepin'." A tall dapper gentleman nearby responds with the slower, Barbra Streisand version: "In the palm of your hand." Oh my God! We are speaking the language of music. And specifically: oldies!

You, sir, are my people!

At checkout, I have a whole recurring joke with this world-weary cashier. We mooooan about the air-conditioning, about prices, her buggy scanner, my stiff joints, we mooooan about moaning. Today, it hits me: she and I share the tongue of collaborative improv comedy. We are speaking Burford!

You, ma'am, must harken from Danville!

Leaving the store with Arlene, I'm exhilarated and emboldened. When we pass a couple teenagers head-bobbing along to some shared music on their earbuds, I bob along too—and they break out into grins. We're not speaking in music; we're speaking in dance!

Kinspeople! Let us share the moves!

All of us have found and lost our "perfect playmates," probably more than once. Yes, we can mourn and miss them. But they've left us with the tools we need to find new playmates, for a moment or forever, wherever and whenever we want.

FIGURE OUT WHO YOU AREN'T

I have never been any good at order and structure. I just don't have an organized mind at all. The way I found that out about myself, ironically enough, was by signing up for the air force during World War II, when I was all of seventeen years old. Not because I wanted to be a pilot, but because I couldn't face being drafted into the army, where I'd have to fight with a gun.

During basic training, the rules were just like West Point. We had to be able to bounce a quarter on our made-up cots every morning. Our pants' creases had to be razor sharp, shoes shined all over, and our trunks organized, with everything perfectly aligned in its place.

You've heard the term *square meals*? Here's what that means: you're literally "at attention" when you eat your meals, back straight up in the chair, legs at a perfect right angle, feet flat and toes pointed straight ahead. Chin up, eyes forward, you cut your food into one little forkable bite at a time, lift your fork straight up out in front of you, then another right angle into your mouth. Like a robot.

Fork food. Arm up. Food in. Arm out. Arm down.

Every single bite, every single meal.

Somehow, all my buddies could do that perfectly. Meanwhile, my "square meal" looked something like this:

Cut food too hard, so it flies off plate. Try again. And again.

Lift first bite with fork. Drop bite. Again and again.

Table and floor covered with food.

Buddies chortle.

Scowls of disapproval from the higher ranks.

My failure wasn't for lack of trying. I struggled with every bone in my body to master the square meal, to keep my pants pressed and my trunk ordered. It was excruciating! But I just couldn't do it.

At a fundamental level, I realized then, I'm not that kind of person. I'm messy, and there's no other word for it.

But here's a twist. All that mistake-making meant a pileup of demerits. And the punishment for every demerit was an hour marching. Which, for me, turned out to be no punishment at all.

Out on the parade grounds, the leading officer barked his orders. Marching in close formation, we were expected to follow along, to keep rigid time with his barks and do everything in perfect sync.

All around me, the other guys struggled. Their pivots were wan and incomplete. They bumbled left instead of right. They staggered trying to keep the rhythm, and with the meager height they could hoist their legs, they'd be lucky to make it over a tiny fallen branch, much less a log.

Meanwhile, in the middle of that mess was me. The officer's barks were making it to my brain as drumbeats, and my long legs were responding in perfect time. What's more—how could this be?—they were soaring upward, easily into a right angle, miles higher than my neighbors'. I had to hold them back to keep them from hitting my chest! When the drumbeat said "pivot," my body pivoted like a door slamming shut. And always in the correct direction.

Why was this so easy?! Why did this feel so . . . natural?!

I barely heard the moaning and groaning all around me, too enthralled with my own achievement. I was loving this! It felt performative and theatrical, like being in a show. In high school musicals, I'd done a bit of basic dancing, but nothing that felt this amazingly right.

Later, sweating in the afterglow, I wondered why my upper body at mealtime couldn't behave like my lower body just had out on the field. Then I realized: my marching had depended on the drumbeat—aka the officer's barks. Square meals didn't come with musical accompaniment, and I felt pretty sure that a metronome wouldn't be allowed at the table.

Oh, well. Own your victory!

One Saturday, my parents made it to the base for their first visiting day, eager to spring me and take me out to lunch. But, by then, I had accumulated a pile of demerits high enough to warrant more weekend marching.

So, rather than not visit with me at all, they brought their lunch to a bench at the edge of the parade grounds, and sat there all afternoon, watching my show. An adoring audience of two. I shouldn't have felt proud, but I really did.

After basic training, it was on to pilot's training, where I flunked my military exams and was deemed an air force failure. Instead, I was reassigned to another division, more suited to my particular abilities: the Special Services, where I would spend the rest of my military career building sets and performing in variety shows.

Theater! Something I'd always loved and been good at. Something that was me. And now I had an extra skill under my belt that might come in handy. Thanks to all those hours on the parade ground, I could really move to a beat!

Going into the air force, I didn't know I was all wrong for a life of rigidity and order. So, I am immensely grateful for that early life lesson. I'm just as grateful to the military for helping me see and appreciate what would later become crucial career assets: good rhythm and a powerful pair of legs.

Finding out who I wasn't showed me who I was.

DON'T LITTER: TIPS FOR SAFETY AND HYGIENE ON FAMILY ROAD TRIPS IN THE 1950S

During the early years of marriage and starting a family, I was still on the road a lot, going from club to club and job to job. A lot of times, I'd bring the family along—my wife Margie and our first kids Chris and Barry, who were very young at the time.

Barry remembers that he and Chris carried all their toys in pillowcases over their shoulders like Santa Claus. As soon as we got into a new motel room, they'd dump them out and play with them for as long as the gig lasted, one or two days usually. Then they'd pack up all their toys and take them to the next night's motel.

They slept in a footlocker in the back of the station wagon so they wouldn't roll around. And when they got too big for that, we put a mattress down back there.

Of course, in those days, we smoked like fiends in the car, often with the windows rolled up. Barry loved the smell of cigarettes when we first lit them, but after that they were awful.

Chris was fascinated with the car's cigarette lighter—you push the button in, it pops out, and you light up, like magic. One day, he was sitting up front between Margie and me, and he tried it himself, pushing the button and waiting for the pop, then bringing the red-hot lighter right up to his mouth . . . where a cigarette was not. He stuck it right in his mouth and burned the hell out of his lips and tongue.

Traveling long stretches across the empty desert, there weren't that many places to stop and change diapers. Instead, we'd change the boys on the road: me driving, holding their legs up, Margie in the passenger seat doing the dirty part. Back then, we had cloth diapers, which were not exactly odor-proof, so you can imagine what that car smelled like.

Eventually, disposable diapers came around, which was a help. Once, Margie had just changed one of the kids, and the diaper stank to high heaven. I could not have it in the car. So, I grabbed it and hurled it out my open window. I didn't need to look—we were in the desert and there hadn't been another car for miles!

Oops. Sure enough, just at that moment, another car had come out of nowhere and was now passing from behind, right into the line of fire. The diaper hit the windshield, smack dead center, splattering its contents all over the glass.

The car braked hard and we shot ahead. I froze for a second and thought: *Should I stop?*

Instead, I floorboarded it and just kept going.

DON'T COUNT ON "THE BIG BREAK"

In 1948, a guy I barely knew from Danville swept back into town and saved me from a sputtering career in advertising. Phil Erickson said: "Let's go to LA," and I said yes!

Since leaving Danville, Phil had been out on the road with a comedy act, but his partner had just ditched him and he needed a replacement. At twenty-one, I had a thin résumé in local theater and Phil had seen me act for less than a single rehearsal. Apparently, though, he saw promise and/or was just plain desperate. Without even an audition, I was hired.

For the next half decade, Phil and I were the Merry Mutes, lip-synching send-ups of the classics and sprinkling in Lewis and Martin–style comedy. We became fast friends, and we had an instant rapport onstage, but it was always a panicked struggle to book our next gig or achieve even a semblance of career momentum. For years, the Merry Mutes were "almost" making it, which meant the families we were struggling to support (Phil had a wife and kids, and my wife Margie and I were planning to have some of our own) were "almost" making it too.

Just a few months into our run in Los Angeles, our comedy was proving a bit lowbrow for the bigger clubs, and we lost a bunch of bookings. Just then, the brand-new medium of television came calling and we jumped at our chance at this bold, new future.

We were booked for a spot on the Don Lee Network, a big radio broadcasting operation that was just getting into TV. Their brand-new headquarters were outside LA, high up on Mount Wilson, which meant a long bumpy ride for Phil and me in my 1935 Ford Phaeton convertible clunker.

True to form, on the final leg of our ascent, the car sputtered, smoked, and then conked out. Our hearts sunk. This was our big break and we were going to miss it because of car trouble.

"No way," Phil said, grabbing all our costumes and props from the back seat. "It can't be that much farther."

And so we hoofed it. And hoofed it and hoofed it.

Finally, the bright lights of the studio were looming above us. Drenched in sweat, we approached the front door, fully expecting to be told we'd missed our slot. By some miracle, we had not!

The studio was blindingly bright and so much more sweltering than the air outside, thanks to an arsenal of massive lights all around us. We worked our sweaty bodies into our costumes as fast as we could, and were hastily slathered in gray makeup, black lipstick, and tons of eyeliner. Otherwise, the crew told us, we'd be practically invisible on the small screen. The medium of television then was all very experimental, before even Kinescope. It was all Phil and I could do not to crack up just looking at each other.

Then, suddenly, we were live! And boy were we ready. Not only had we honed our little act onstage, we had also done our homework on performing for TV: huddled around Phil's little seven-inch set watching Milton Berle, we realized that comedy needed to be big and physical to register on-screen. So, we took our broad, hokey act and made it even broader and hokier! Judging by the grinning crew members squinting into their little monitor, it was working!

Our segment was over before we knew it, and we let ourselves breathe. This was live TV, no recording, so it was not exactly clear who out there in the world might have caught the Merry Mutes' small-screen debut. We hoped and imagined maybe someone important.

Minutes later, Phil and I staggered out of that inferno and took in the mountain air, a pair of soggy, gray-faced crazies with big, black-lipped grins. We laughed at each other and with each other, and rejoiced in our milestone moment.

We were part of the future, even if we didn't have a car.

Well, I guess nobody that important caught the show, because Phil and I returned unceremoniously to our life of barely getting by. Eventually, we took our act on the road, out into the desert and across the country, with more automotive mishaps, sparsely attended gigs, humiliation, and self-doubt. One night when this Mute was feeling particularly unmerry, a kind out-of-the-blue pep talk from the future king of showbiz himself, Liberace, put the wind back in my sails and kept me giving my all to the act.

In 1949, Phil and I landed our dream of a stable gig in Atlanta—two shows a day at the Henry Grady Hotel—and decided to settle there with our young families. During our time off, we honed our act on the radio and at all sorts of local events.

One day, television called again, and not the late-night local variety either. This was the call that every up-and-coming performer dreams of: a booking on Ed Sullivan's huge popular national TV talent showcase, *Toast of the Town*.

Here it was, finally, a *real* chance to break into the big time!

Both of us were elated, and when we delivered the good news to our wives, friends, and coworkers, we reveled in their astonished excitement. In their eyes, and in our own, we were finally *somebodies.*

We went into overdrive rehearsing our best bits—we only had two minutes on air, so we really had to nail every second—then flew up to New York to do the program. Turns out we were booked for the same show as Margaret Truman, the daughter of President Harry Truman, who was working hard on her own budding career as an opera singer.

So far, she'd been getting some very mixed reviews for her talent, most famously in a 1950 *Washington Post* story that said: "She is flat a good deal of the time. And she cannot sing with anything approaching professional finish." That earned the critic a violent note from Margaret's protective father, the president himself, that quickly became national news: "Someday I hope to meet you. When that happens, you'll need a new nose, a lot of beefsteak for black eyes, and perhaps a supporter below!"

We listened from backstage as Margaret went on first, and I can't say the critic was wrong. *At least we don't have a tough act to follow*, we thought.

But then came the audience applause. They were roaring and calling for an encore! Which had never happened on live TV before, but guess what? They granted Margaret Truman an encore.

Phil and I looked at each other, and both our faces dropped at the same moment. We realized what this meant for our act—the very same thing we'd feared after our Mount Wilson breakdown.

This was live TV and the schedule was strict. Our two minutes were being swallowed up by the president's daughter.

We listened dejectedly as yet another round of applause filled the studio, and by the time a sheepish producer finally came over to officially deliver the bad news, our hearts were well broken.

There may have been a vague plan of rebooking us, but I don't remember, and it never materialized anyway. Feeling again like miserable failures, we headed back to Atlanta, dreading having to face all those people who had tuned in eagerly to delight in our big break.

I worried that the writing was on the wall for the Merry Mutes, though I could never admit it to Phil. Maybe our big break would never come! Indeed it didn't, and after a few more years in Atlanta, we went our separate ways.

The Margaret Truman Incident still stings today. To have our hopes dashed, right at their highest, was the cruelest of cruelties. But between this experience and our post–Don Lee fizzle years earlier, I did learn a lesson that would come in handy for surviving all the lost jobs and mothballed projects in my future: there's no such thing as a sure thing.

HONE YOUR BIT (EVERY JOB IS TRAINING FOR THE NEXT ONE)

Tie flapping and microphone in hand, I scampered over the French Quarter's cobblestones and claimed the spot for my on-camera report: a corner with a big crowd gathered behind me, their attention focused farther up the street. My camera crew caught up and readied the shot, just in time.

It was 1955 and I was hustling hard in New Orleans television. I had an eight-hour stint as announcer, but that's not why I cared about the job. In the afternoons, I also had my own little comedy-variety show. And for that, it was time to pull out the character I'd happened upon during my high school magic act mishap: the suave, supremely confident buffoon.

"It's a beautiful Sunday here in the Quarter, and the ladies of the Krewe of Venus are rolling our way! This year, we're told, the Venus parade will tell the story of *the ballet*! Expect arabesques! Expect pirouettes! In just a few seconds, we'll get the perfect view of their first float! And here they come now!!"

With that, I turned excitedly, and the Venus parade, which behind me had gotten extremely close, abruptly turned a corner and headed off down a different street. From where I had positioned us, on purpose, the camera couldn't capture a thing, except for the back of onlookers' heads and maybe a sliver of a float.

I stood there for a second, acting flat-footed, giving the camera my best little momentary panicked face of *Oops*. Then, just as quickly, I shot into recovery mode, pointing wildly to something off camera and urging the cameraman to follow.

The shot lurched, and there, out in the middle of the empty street, a stray cat had stopped to scratch itself. My ideal scene partner.

"Now, who do we have here?!" I cooed.

Noting the attention, the cat crouched defensively.

"Will you look at that!" I fawned gaspingly. "A perfect plié!"

In New Orleans, there's a Mardi Gras parade every other minute, so I kept this hapless on-the-street reporter bit going day after day, for as long as I could make it funny. The first couple times, I was told later, my Louisiana audience thought I was actually that bad. Then, once they got the joke, they tuned in religiously for its next iteration.

DON'T DO LIVE MORNING TV

Later in 1955, I got my first big gig on national TV, hosting CBS's *The Morning Show*! For the first time in a career of constant scrambling, it was steady, well-paid work, and my wife Margie and I could breathe a sigh of relief.

But on my very first day on the job, my car blew up in the driveway—what is it with me and big breaks and breakdowns?! Jumping into the unlucky commuter's plan B, I took a quick taxi to the train, then another much slower taxi to the studio, arriving fifteen minutes late—to a live broadcast! That pretty much set the tone for my year on the show.

Every morning, five days a week, we did an hour and a half show for the East Coast, then repeated the exact same show for the West Coast—three full hours of live TV. I was up against NBC's *Today* with Dave Garroway, who was very popular, so nobody on either coast ever saw me. For those few who did tune in, here's what they would have caught:

Me trying to cover for slurring drunk jazz musicians still up from their gigs the night before.

A pack of Canadian sled dogs tearing down three sets, all because, during my interview with the sled driver, I just couldn't stop myself from saying "mush," which is sled dog for "go."

And perhaps the strangest interview I ever did, with the French indoor tennis champion Pierre Etchebaster. Before the show, he came to me and said: "I don't want any reading of those cue cards. Let's just talk." Well, that sounded refreshing. "Okay!" I said.

But as soon as we were live, I introduced him and he promptly got out of his seat, walked straight over to the camera and stuck his face in the lens, like a millimeter from the glass. *What was going on?!* I had to beg him to come back and sit down for the interview, but when he finally did, he wouldn't say a word. Not a word. So I had to do the whole interview myself, with him just sitting there, silently staring into the camera.

"I hope I pronounced your last name correctly?"

"I imagine there's differences between indoor tennis and the outdoor variety?"

"Smaller courts maybe."

"What happens if the ball hits the ceiling?"

Tick . . . tick . . . tick . . .

When you're "just talking" to yourself, two minutes feels like all five centuries of the Dark Ages.

SOME SECRETS YOU SHOULDN'T TELL

One of my favorite segments of my CBS morning show was storytelling time. As a dad, I'd grown to love making up bedtime tales for my kids, fine-tuning the funny bits and the dramatic turning points night after night. Storytelling time on the show was kind of like that, only bright and early in the morning and with millions of kids as my audience.

For each segment, I would do modern updates of the old fairy-tale classics like the Brothers Grimm and Hans Christian Andersen, telling the story and acting out the parts. At the same time, I was drawing it for the audience too. I'd use a pen to sketch a picture of the part I was reading on a big easel, then flip the page and do a new sketch for the next part.

People used to marvel at how I could draw so perfectly, while talking and acting at the same time, on national television. Each one of those illustrations was incredible.

Well, here's my secret. Television back then was black and white, and there's one color that doesn't show up in black and white at all. Blue. It's just invisible. Which was a real problem for people with blue eyes: on TV, they'd look like aliens, their eyes just totally blocked out.

With storytelling time, this technological limitation worked to my advantage. Before each show, I would carefully draw out all the illustrations with a blue pen. To the home audience, the pages looked blank when I first started. But in the studio, I could see all those blue lines perfectly. And so, I'd just trace them!

You couldn't get away with that now, not with color.

I told this story to my adult son Barry the other day and he just looked at me, stunned. As a little kid, he'd watched my storytelling segment in the mornings too.

"I never knew you did that," he said. "All these years, I never knew."

EGGS AGAIN? SOME FAILURES ARE JUST THAT

Years after my failed but transformative magic trick in high school assembly, eggy embarrassment struck again. But this time, nothing good came out of it at all. Except, I suppose, this story.

In 1958, having been canned from CBS just three years into a ten-year contract, I found myself again in the "take whatever work you can get" phase of my career. Thus, here I was hosting a game show called *Mother's Day*, which pitted real mothers against one another in quizzes and contests that tested their homemaking skills and maternal know-how. I gave it my all, but the show was awful.

On one episode, the contestants were challenged with telling the difference between a raw egg and a hard-boiled one. After they did all their testing and inspecting and choosing, it was my job to crack the eggs they'd chosen as hard-boiled into a pan. Two mothers' eggs were raw, but there was one lucky winner. When it came time to explain to the audience how you can tell the difference, I brought out two eggs of my own.

"I'll show you how to tell an egg," I began, which made no sense whatsoever and sent me right off the tracks. "You spin it," I continued, spinning one egg and then another, regaining steam. "See, one spins more than the other. Now I'll show you the hard-boiled egg." With that, I confidently cracked what I thought to be the cooked egg into the pan.

Splat! My stomach twisted, and after some chuckling and forehead-palming, I attempted to recover: "The hard-boiled egg spins faster. One did spin faster, didn't it? I probably picked up the wrong egg. But I know! I know!"

It was as if I had learned nothing from my teenage egg mishap! Instead of grandly rolling with failure, I tried to claw my way out of it. I let them see me sweat!

Some humiliations never die. On my ninety-ninth birthday that clip resurfaced on the internet. Until then, I had successfully forgotten it.

DANCE WITH CHITA

Like most of us, I've had precious times in life or work when things just go perfectly smoothly. Performing alongside my son Barry in *Diagnosis: Murder*—a daily joy. A spontaneous sailing trip in the Virgin Islands with my beloved partner Michelle in the early 1980s, days and days with the wind just right, gliding us over the warm Caribbean.

These times, I often told myself, felt just like dancing with Chita. Chita being Chita Rivera, my costar in the Broadway musical *Bye Bye Birdie* back in the early 1960s.

The more I think about it now, though, this analogy gives short shrift to what was most important about both my relationship with Chita and navigating life in general. *Perfectly smooth*, I have come to see, doesn't mean easy at all.

Before I was cast in *Bye Bye Birdie*, I was a total nobody on the Great White Way. I had three years of TV at CBS, a failed pilot, and after months of desperate pavement-pounding, a single short-lived supporting chorus role under my belt. Plus: zero dance training and a barely passable singing voice. I wasn't ready for Broadway and I didn't feel ready, and I only landed the audition for *Bye Bye Birdie* because a well-connected producer convinced the director to take a chance on me.

Meanwhile, Chita had already broken out big as Anita in *West Side Story*, Broadway's megahit of all megahits. That meant now she had her pick of projects. When producers approached her for the role in *Bye Bye Birdie*, somebody else told her the show was total garbage, so she and her agent concocted a way to politely brush off the offer. But then Chita went in to hear the music for herself, fell in love, and said she had to do it, leaving her agent stunned.

All of which is to say that Chita came to the show with the wind in her sails, and I felt like a stowaway.

But boy, did she have a way of making me feel like I belonged on board, from the get-go. On the first day of rehearsals, we bonded instantly as fellow goofballs, which put me right at ease. And from that place of connection and safety, I was able to take up the task of learning all that goes into a Broadway role.

Chita, my more seasoned castmates, our generous director Gower Champion, always true to his name—these were all my teachers. I took in way more than the technical stuff like dance and vocal training. Each day was one other explosive lesson in performance after another: building a character arc, layering comedy and emotion into my singing, all the ways of working with a live audience. Much later, remembering this experience, Chita told me: "We all watched you. You sucked it all up and gave it all out."

With Chita specifically, we had real chemistry and trust, which gave us the freedom, in our scenes and numbers together, to experiment, surprise one another, make each moment crackly and fresh.

In rehearsals, our "failures" were sheer joy. During one scene, Chita's character Rose is really mad at me, Albert, and her line was: "You go your way and I'll go my way, east and west on the Lincoln Highway." Which made no sense to me at all, and so I looked at Chita, utterly lost. She didn't know what it meant either, which was written all over her face.

I cracked up, and then she cracked up and eventually, Gower just told us to go home.

As for our dancing, getting the steps down was just my foundation. Chita showed me the musical and emotional power in every part of the human body: hips, shoulders, chin, wrists.

At first, all I could do was follow her, and I did it fairly well. But there was always this look in her eye telling me: "Show me *you*. Do it *your* way." And as soon as I did, I could feel her practically nodding "yes, yes!" And then taking us even further!

When we finally opened, we were a well-oiled machine. Night after night, for over a year of performances, Chita Rivera made me feel like Fred Astaire.

Like every show, ours had its technical issues. For instance, one night at the end of "How to Kill a Man," one of the two wires holding me high above the stage snapped, leaving me dangling and spinning and praying for my life (rest assured, my prayers were answered).

But in performance with Chita, there was no such thing as flailing.

Sometimes, she would get downstage of me and make faces to try and break me up. Sure, she was having a bit of fun with me because I was so green. But she was also reminding me that we weren't just performing what we'd rehearsed; we were live and real together, and in that moment, anything could happen. The energy that gave me was exhilarating.

And that prepared me for the onstage experience, which I now realize is the truest manifestation of "dancing with Chita."

The final scene of *Bye Bye Birdie* is not some big, rousing full-cast number. It's "Rosie," a quiet, sweet love song-and-dance set at a train depot, where the on-again, off-again romance between Rose and Albert (Chita and Dick) is finally on again, for good. It's a long, leisurely number: this is our time to really play together, happy at last.

Well, one particular night, we took *play* to a whole new level. Most of the number went off as usual: Chita and I sang and frolicked around the benches, I whisked her around on a luggage cart, we danced side by side and slapped our knees in time, we waltzed, we spun . . .

And then, nearing the song's finale together, we moved in for an embrace—and somehow, do not ask me how—the buckles on Chita's big belt and my belt got stuck together.

In both of our eyes, we saw the realization hit.

First, we tried to pry apart delicately, still singing.

Uh-oh—still stuck.

A little harder—still stuck.

Then, it hit us: we were in this moment, live, together. Of course, we must go with it!

Letting the audience in on our little snafu, we started twisting and tugging more dramatically, back and forth. We let our little dilemma wash over our facial expressions, really getting into the frustration.

And the crowd was right there with us, laughing hysterically. A mistake! Live onstage! This is what theater audiences crave!

Well, what happened next took it right over the top: somehow, in our struggle to disentangle, we both lost our balance, then our belts broke free, sending both us—each in our own way—falling. Fully. On the stage. Side by side, right on our butts!

Now the crowd was roaring and clapping.

Meanwhile, the orchestra was repeating and stalling for us, hoping against hope that we might recover to finish the number.

And we did! We leaped back onto our feet together, nodded briefly to the audience to "thank" them for appreciating our foolishness, then joined hands to wrap up the number, grinning and glowing in the aftermath.

Now I'd had a few graceful recoveries in the past (ahem, Egg Trick), but to share this one with another person, with Chita, was existentially transcendent. All that trust we'd built together, that muscle we'd developed to embrace the unexpected, to stay in and go with the moment, all of that had been training for this: our chance to face disaster, as one, and spin it into triumph.

That, my friends, is the real definition of "life going smoothly."

GO NUTS (BUT MAYBE NOT *THAT* NUTS)

One day on the set of *The Dick Van Dyke Show*, Carl presented the cast with a draft script for an upcoming episode, "It May Look Like a Walnut." We had been part of its gestation, as always, so we thought we knew what to expect. Then we all started reading. And gasping. And squealing with laughter. The writers had made it their mission to surprise us, and they had succeeded.

The script starts at night with Rob glued to a terrifying movie on TV about a band of creepy aliens taking over Earth. Laura begs him to stop watching, covering her head in pillows, desperate to block it out.

Rather than let her rest, Rob insists on regaling her with the movie's eeriest details: the aliens have no thumbs and extra eyes in the back of their heads, they subsist on walnuts, and their leader is a Danny Thomas lookalike.

The next morning, all is well for Rob, until details of the movie start coming to life all around him. Laura makes walnuts for breakfast. Danny Thomas appears at the office—with no thumbs and eyes in the back of his head. Back at home, Laura sprouts eyes in the back of her head too! And in the climax of Rob's living nightmare, he opens a closet door and out cascades an avalanche of walnuts with a gleeful Laura bodysurfing on top of them.

Two seasons in, we had sprinkled in moments of absurdity in prior episodes, but nothing like this. The nightmare walnut gag was extended through the entire episode, never letting up, only getting bigger and weirder. The writers were pushing the needle on TV comedy with the script, and the whole cast was thrilled to meet the challenge they'd laid at our feet.

Outside our little bubble, however, there were powerful skeptics. When our executive producer, Sheldon Leonard, and network higher-ups read the script, they despised it. "Too bizarre," they complained to Carl. "It's science fiction, not comedy." Their only note on the script was to kill it.

But Carl, who trusted his writers and our reactions, pushed back. "Bizarre" was the whole point, he explained patiently to the naysayers. If we commit to the unrelenting outlandishness, the audience would be right there with us, laughing harder and harder.

Eventually, the higher-ups wearied of their fight with Carl and relented, though I'm pretty sure they still thought we'd all lost their minds.

On the first day of rehearsal, a ton of walnuts arrived on set, and we all rejoiced. "Over-the-top weird" was even more hilarious in the flesh than it had been on the page.

Rather quickly, though, the joke began turning against us. The nut wholesaler had delivered far more walnuts than was needed to fill that closet, so for the whole week of rehearsals, piles of extra walnuts sat around the set. Naturally, the cast and crew started cracking them open and eating them.

At first, they were tasty and satisfying, a fun little change of pace from our usual on-set snack fare. But then we kept eating them . . . and eating and eating and eating them. No longer because we enjoyed them; just because they were there.

First came the stomachaches. Then the bloating, gas, and constipation. Walnuts, you see, are very high in fiber and fat. And an excess of the two can wreak all sorts of havoc on the digestive system. By the end of the week, we had a mass case of gastric distress.

And the fun doesn't stop there. The night after we taped the show, we all staggered out into the studio parking lot, doubled-over and eager to get home to our private bathrooms. Instead, for me alone, fresh horror awaited. When I reached for the door handle of my car, a two-seater convertible Jaguar XKE, I saw that its entire interior was filled to the brim . . . with *walnuts*. As everyone else drove away, I just stood there, letting it sink in. Some wise guys had decided to up the ante on the walnut gag yet again, in real life!

Objectively, one might admire the prank for its sheer audacity. I, however, was not objective. I cursed the culprits, whoever they were, then opened my door to release the walnuts. Unlike the satisfying cascade from the closet that we'd just filmed, however, the spillage from my car was minimal. With both doors open, I hadn't even gotten rid of half of those things! I reached in and started shoveling, but at that rate, I realized I'd be at it all night.

I gave up and stomped back into the studio to find another ride home.

By Monday, everyone was regular again and chortling over the prank, except for me. I'd spent the whole weekend ridding my car of those walnuts! The only meager revenge I had against the culprits was refusing them the satisfaction of figuring out who they were.

Their "joke" kept giving for months to come too. I'd open the glovebox and a confetti of white walnut meat would flutter out. I'd put up the top and get a shower of shells. Something would slide under the seat, and when I reached to retrieve it, my knuckles would scrape on you-know-what. My foot would detect a little snag of resistance from the gas pedal or the brake, and I'd curse out loud.

"It May Look Like a Walnut" turned out to be one of our most popular episodes, proving those narrow-minded execs wrong and Carl's creative instincts correct, which emboldened us all to take more comedic risks in episodes to come, and in our careers after the show. To this day, though, don't even show me a walnut! I will not laugh.

SUCK UP TO THE LANDLADY

Like a lot of TV shows in the 1960s, *The Dick Van Dyke Show* was filmed in rented space at Desilu-Cahuenga Studios. This was one of the properties of Desilu Productions, founded and run by Lucille Ball and Desi Arnaz, which Lucy took over in 1962 after they divorced. This made her the most powerful woman in the business.

Once she took charge, Lucy made a point of making the rounds and keeping up with goings-on at the various shows filming at her studios. The first time she popped in on us was quite a surprise: during rehearsal, we heard a cackle from up on the catwalk, and there she was, enjoying the show. At first, the cast was all rattled, like we'd been caught at something.

But our producer Carl Reiner, who already knew Lucy, broke the ice and we quickly realized how friendly and kind she was. We were always having fun on that set, and when Lucy came by, she seemed to enjoy getting in on the fun, even if it was just for a minute.

I also must admit that I wanted her to like me, so I tried extra hard to be funny when she was around. One day, I came up with a rather obvious gag on the spot, which was that she was the landlady letting the place fall to pieces, and I was the disgruntled tenant.

"Um, Miss Ball, there's a layer of dust all over these rafters here, and it's giving me horrible allergies."

"Miss Ball, what kind of establishment are you running here? The trash cans are overflowing!"

In retrospect, she may have found this insulting. But if she did, she didn't show it. No, Lucy played along and kept it going until we both got bored.

"I'm so sorry, Mr. Van Dyke, I'll get the cleaners out here right away."

"Carl! Take out the trash! Why is it so hard to get a decent janitor!"

From there, Lucy and I fell into a long friendship, with much improvement in our shared comedy. When she guest starred on my comedy-variety show *Van Dyke and Company*, a decade later, we sang, we danced, she punched me over a couch, poured coffee in my lap, broke a bottle over my head, pushed me off a balcony in a wheelchair, and shocked me in the mouth with an exposed electrical wire.

SPEAK UP FOR YOUR FAMILY

Carl Reiner was a friend and hero for too many reasons to count.

One of which is that he was a fighter. During our years working together, he consistently went to the mat for the show against the higher-ups. He spoke up for our writers and actors and protected us like a father.

I've told you about the walnut episode, when Carl stuck up for our comedy. To me, his more important battles were against the network's uptight, hypocritical moralism. Some of those he won and some he lost, but they were all worth it.

Most famously, he pushed for Rob and Laurie Petrie to sleep in the same bed, like pretty much every other married couple in America in the 1960s. Standards and Practices told him it was in bad taste, and so we stayed trapped in our silly little twin beds for the show's entire run.

He had more success backing up Mary Tyler Moore's desire to wear—gasp!—capri pants!

The network hated an episode about Rob's maternity ward "baby switch" panic for too many reasons to count, none of which made sense. When the audience finally meets the father of the baby Rob assumes has been switched with his own, Rob (and we) see that man is Black. First the executives chafed that we were making the Black man the butt of the joke. Then when Carl explained that, no, the joke was on Rob, the paranoid white guy, they hated the episode even more. Fortunately, Carl won that skirmish, too, and it turned out to be one of the most popular episodes of the whole run.

Carl's good fight didn't end with our first series together either.

In the early 1970s, he produced, and I starred in another family sitcom *The New Dick Van Dyke Show.* Sybil Adelman wrote a script where the daughter character walks into her parents' bedroom while they're having sex (off camera, don't worry).

The episode deals with the comic fallout: the parents anxiously struggle to figure out why their daughter is suddenly acting so weird, then, when they figure out what she saw, they sit down with her to gently explain it. The show handled the situation, one an awful lot of parents have found themselves in, with matter-of-fact honesty, and we were all proud of it.

CBS went nuts and absolutely refused to air the episode in the US. Meanwhile, it ran in Canada and nobody died.

Again, Carl stood up for his writers, very publicly. He pointed out that the network allowed all sorts of "risqué" material on its other shows, e.g., Norman Lear's *All in the Family* (menopause) and *Maude* (abortion). He even threatened to leave the show if the network didn't back down. In fighting for what he knew to be right, even if it came at great personal cost, Carl set an example that none of us would forget.

The response from CBS still gets me fuming today. Network president Robert Wood told *The New York Times* that the episode was "out of rhythm with the tradition of Dick Van Dyke's kind of entertainment."

"Audiences bring a certain level of expectancy to all programs," he went on. "With 'All in the Family' there is a certain expectation that the topic might be menopause, but Dick Van Dyke has wholesome written all over his face and is remembered by people for his Walt Disney roles."

The gall. Not only were they censoring us, they were using my "wholesome" image as their cudgel to do it! Let me tell you: I cultivated my family-friendly image deliberately, and there was nothing in that subject matter that stood in tension with my image. Talking with your kids about difficult stuff is the very definition of family-friendly.

Carl made good on his threat and there was no way I was going to continue without him. So, with great disgust, I threw in the towel too.

I really wish this story was ancient history. But, as I'm sure you know, censorship in the name of "family-friendly" has made a very big comeback in recent years. I won't get on a soapbox and depress you with a litany of examples you probably already know. But I will say this: real family values are not the exclusive property of one political persuasion over another. Nor do they belong to one kind of family over another. Unfortunately, though, a lot of people in power don't see it that way. Which means the world needs a lot more Carl Reiners right now, voices and leaders who stick up not just for a select few, but for all of us.

IT DOESN'T TAKE A GOOD BOSS TO DO GREAT WORK

Not every workplace has a Carl Reiner in charge, which can make it challenging to do a good job. But not impossible.

A quick warning: I'm starting this one off on a tart note, but I do have a good reason for it.

I've made no secret about my less-than-great impressions of the directors of the two movies I am most famous for. About all the *Mary Poppins* director gave us actors was: "Action. Cut. Now another one just like that." Stiff and uninspiring. *Chitty Chitty Bang Bang*'s director was a playboy vulgarian (and not just because it's a play on Vulgaria, from the movie) who loathed children, trudged through the job, and admitted freely that the only reason he was doing the picture at all was so he could buy a Rolls-Royce.

When you think about it, it's truly astounding. Two of the most beloved movies for kids in history were directed by a couple of total sourpusses.

I know they were very good at setting up shots and editing and everything, but when it came to bringing out great performances in their actors, they just weren't there. And more broadly, in bringing alive the real beating heart of those movies, the things that make them unforgettable and classic, that stuff wasn't the directors' doing at all.

The people we can thank for that, *in spite of* who they were working under, are the exquisite artists who created the music and dancing.

When Walt Disney sat me down with the songwriting duo Robert and Richard Sherman to hear what they'd come up with for *Mary Poppins*, I wept at their performance. There was so much warmth and textured character in their melodies and lyrics, it felt the Shermans had rolled out a full emotional blueprint for me to bring Bert the Chimney Sweep alive.

Most people recall the chorus of "Chim Chim Cher-ee," but not much else. It's an ode to the world of the lowly chimney sweep of Victorian London, with an aching tension between chipper lyrics and a minor key. When I, as Bert, sing to the two Banks children staring up their chimney, the song tingles with a kind of spiritual awe.

Up where the smoke
Is all billered and curled
'Tween pavement and stars
Is the chimney sweep world

In the movie, I felt that awe as I sang, and you can see it on the faces of me and my castmates. It could have been a throwaway "soft moment" in the number, but thanks to the lyrics and music, it was a revelation.

The Shermans' music had the exact same effect on Julie Andrews. Their songs made no-nonsense Mary Poppins three-dimensional, surprisingly playful and tender.

Inspired by the musical gift they'd laid at her feet, Julie poured her soul into the melancholy lullaby "Feed the Birds," a heartrending plea for kindness and compassion. That song was Walt's favorite, and for many of us on set, it became the beating heart of the entire movie, a mood and spirit to aspire to in all of our work.

And who could forget "Supercalifragilisticexpialidocious"?! In rehearsing and filming that number day after day, the music let Julie, me, our young costars, and all the extras just wallow in silly childhood fun.

When I got the offer for my next movie, *Chitty Chitty Bang Bang*, I would have turned it down had the Sherman brothers not been hired to do the music. I was worried that the movie would be all about gadgetry and special effects, but Robert and Richard's work tugged the spotlight back where it belonged: on the humans.

Filming the title number, the prop car got most of the director's attention, but that's not why we, the cast, were bouncing in our seats. All our joy came from playing together with those delicious rhythms and words.

My favorite song was "You Two," in which my character, a widowed inventor, celebrates his unique, single-dad bond with his kids over breakfast. Under the song's ostensible cheer, the Shermans layered just the faintest hint of grief for the family member not at the table. During filming, we had to contend with another show-stealing contraption (which I'll tell you about later), but it was the music that kept us all connected to what mattered most in the scene.

Richard and Robert's music wasn't the only thing that brought these movies to life for me and the cast. There was also the work of another genius duo, two of my dearest friends.

At the time of *Mary Poppins*, choreographers (and spouses) Dee Dee Wood and Marc Breaux had done some TV work, but their career together was just getting started. They choreographed a dance number for me on *The Dick Van Dyke Show*, and we clicked in a rare way. So, when Walt asked me for recommendations for a choreographer for *Mary Poppins*, their names leaped out of my mouth.

What we all saw happen with Marc and Dee Dee on the set of that movie was breathtaking. This was their first big break, and it was like a dam of creativity just exploding inside them and between them. The spirit they brought to dance seemed to be: Anything is possible! And all of us—from the actors and dancers to the set designers and prop-makers—took that energy and ran with it.

Watch "Step in Time," the epic rooftop chimney sweep number and you'll see what I mean. It features thirty dancers, doing every bit of acrobatic dancing you can imagine—leaps, rolls, back rolls, cartwheels, broom-jumping, prancing on parapets, upside-down hand-walking between two buildings, and that's not even the half of it. From the rooftop, the dancers plummet down the chimney and continue the fun inside the Banks' home, then out into the street.

Describing their work for Rose Eichenbaum's *Masters of Movement: Portraits of America's Great Choreographers*, Dee Dee put it beautifully: "[W]e just took life and translated it into energy, character, and emotion."

Given the number's audacious complexity—it ran twelve minutes long!—it's no surprise that rehearsals took forever. Walt Disney was so in love with the number that he showed up every day to watch it take shape.

Before we started filming, however, the director, true to his mirthless character, whined it was too long and insisted it be cut down to something like two minutes!

To his eternal credit, Walt stepped in, using incredible rehearsal footage to make his case that the number was something special. And for good measure, he suggested adding even more stunts to the dance! So, in the end, it stayed long and stayed in.

Marc and Dee Dee's work on *Chitty Chitty Bang Bang* was just as magnificent, and just as exhausting. In "Me Ol' Bamboo," we danced, spun, and leaped over bamboo sticks at breakneck speed. It took twenty-three takes for all of us to nail it the whole way through.

Today, I watch these movies and still gasp at what these two pairs of artists created. If you ever needed proof that song and dance can transform one's soul, here it is.

My takeaway rule for you, then, is this: Unfortunately, there are a lot of mediocre bosses and leaders out there, but we can't let their mediocrity drag us down. If you can find people who inspire you, who make you feel like you can do your best, then tap into and work off that energy. Together, you can get the whole world singing a brand-new, very long made-up word! Together, you can turn life into energy, character, and emotion!

ACCEPT YOUR LIMITATIONS

I have taken it on the chin for six decades for my godawful Cockney accent in *Mary Poppins*. Over the years, I have accumulated a million different excuses. Here are the top three:

1. I had just one hour with a Cockney dialect coach . . . an Irishman named Pat O'Malley.
2. I was surrounded by a cast of real Brits, none of whom pulled me aside and said: "Um, maybe you should brush up that accent." So, if anything, I blame England for being too polite.
3. I wasn't doing a Cockney accent at all. My character Bert was, in fact, from the very north of England in a shire settled by people from Ohio.

Here's the plain truth: I tried. I really, really tried. But I had a lot more on my plate than just an accent. I had two different roles, a half dozen songs, and lots of very tricky dancing. Maybe all this focus on my Cockney is a little in the weeds?

In *Chitty Chitty Bang Bang*, I tried an accent again, briefly. During my first scene in the movie, when I'm testing my exploding rocket suit, I did some sort of British accent for a few lines:

"Stand bick! Keep cleaah!"

But I quickly realized I sounded ridiculous and there was no way I could possibly keep contorting my mouth and voice like that for the whole rest of the shoot.

"Enough of that," I said to the director after we'd finished the scene. "Can my character please be American?"

A little while after *Mary Poppins*, it was announced that Sean Connery was retiring from his role as James Bond, and they needed a new guy. *Bond* (and *Chitty*) producer Cubby Broccoli called me up and offered me the part.

"Have you heard my British accent?" I replied.

Click.

True story, simplified for efficiency of course.

I would have made a pretty good Bond. A lighter Bond with some comedy. I could have done it a little like Inspector Clouseau, maybe even some singing and dancing. But, fresh off one bad accent, I couldn't stomach the possibility of another.

Only four decades later did I dare try an English accent again. To prep for my part as an old British banker in 2018's *Mary Poppins Returns*, I had a dialectician handcuffed to me, polishing my every syllable.

You can watch for yourself to see how well I acquitted myself in the accent department. But even if I *can* do a passable posh, I'll never try Cockney again.

WIN AN OSCAR

Have you seen my Oscar?

Well, it's not an official one, but to me, it's even better. When Julie Andrews won the Academy Award for *Mary Poppins*, the crew decided I deserved an award myself.

It's a figure of me, or rather my character Bert the Chimney Sweep made of soldered-together scrap metal. Brass I think, judging by the color, which has faded some over the years. It's got a big cylinder head, maybe one of those things a plumber uses to connect pipes?

And it's really got my posture: spindly arms and legs, and a long bendy body, leaning forward into my wire-brush broom. It looks just like I'm in the middle of dancing!

Down at my feet there are metal nuts (as in the partners of bolts), stacked and scattered, and behind me is a star-filled backdrop.

There's a plaque on the stand that reads:

SPECIAL AWARD TO
DICK VAN DYKE
FOR BEING

SUPERCALIFRAGILISTICEXPIALIDOCIOUS
PRESENTED BY
THE "*MARY POPPINS*" PRODUCTION CREW 1965

It was delivered to me at home, I believe, and when I first pulled it out of its box, I was beside myself with delight. Tickled to death and beyond. We all had a ball making that movie together, and this thing just captures that spirit perfectly.

Plus, what an incredible honor—to have people you've worked with create a "thank-you" present with their own hands! Putting so much time and creativity into imagining and tweaking every little detail! For me, this gift was something so rare: an embodiment of pure love. It is my favorite award and whenever I see it over there, all those good feelings come flooding back.

Every time we get evacuated for fires, my "Oscar" is at the top of the list of things to carry out with us. After we fled the Woolsey Fire, Arlene got a great picture of the Oscar and our cat Mooshi, temporarily relocated to her mom's house in Huntington Beach, both waiting to go back home.

I'm sure Julie has her own well-deserved Oscar in a place of honor, but eighty-six actors and seventy-nine actresses have that exact same one. Mine is a one of a kind.

STAY ON THE PHONE

One night in the early 1960s, Cary Grant called me up out of the blue to tell me about LSD. We'd had a friendship of sorts for years, ever since he popped into my dressing room after a show of *Bye Bye Birdie*, perused my wardrobe, and complimented my fashion sense.

But this time was very different.

Along with other Hollywood folks at the time, Cary had been doing guided LSD trips as a psychiatric treatment for years, and he'd been quite public about how much they'd helped. He'd been able to see the connection between his childhood abandonment issues and his three failed marriages, and to liberate himself from his more destructive patterns. "I got where I wanted to go," he would later write, "not completely, because you cut back the barnacles and find more barnacles, and you have to get these off. In life there is no end to getting well."

Judging by his call to me, he was indeed still finding more barnacles. He kept me on the phone for an hour.

I remember he sounded a bit metaphysical, talking about how we were all connected by the particles that make us up. And he told me some freakish details of what he'd seen on his trips, but those I haven't held on to.

What struck me wasn't so much his words, but what was underneath them. There was a sadness in his voice, and urgency, so unlike the charming, clever fellow I thought I'd known. I sensed he was in bad shape.

So, I just kept listening, sitting there in my dark Encino living room with my whole family asleep in the house around me, imagining Cary pacing around in one of his empty spreads. I don't think I got too many words in myself, because he just seemed like he needed to gush.

To this day, I have no idea what was in Cary's head when he picked up the phone and decided to dial my number. I was flattered he had picked me to call and glad that it seemed to help. After that first conversation, Cary started calling regularly. And it was the same pattern. Sometimes he just regaled me with movie-star gossip, which I didn't keep much track of and found mildly entertaining. I remember him telling me he'd just gotten to play the part of a beach bum down in Jamaica, a life that sounded kind of great to both of us. He had career doubts, too, wondering if he should hang up his hat.

I was mostly silent, offering my bits of advice if there was a pause, mostly, again, listening for what he wasn't saying. I felt a little like a priest, waiting for his reluctant confessant to get to the meat of things. At times, it sounded like Cary was thinking of us as kindred spirits, which was touching. But I'd barely said four sentences, so it felt like he was putting something on me that wasn't about me.

Eventually, his calls became about a movie he wanted me to make with him, a Western or a romantic comedy, I can't remember. This territory was more fun for me, and we batted around the idea with easy enthusiasm.

I can't remember when or how these calls from Cary stopped. The movie, whatever it was or was not, never came to pass. In 1966, he retired from the business to raise his daughter and never made another film again.

Like I said, I'd be veering into wild speculation to guess all that was in Cary's head when he made those calls. But as I felt it, here was a friend in a mess that just needed someone to listen. I didn't help him fix any problems, but I also didn't hang up on him mid-ramble. I was a safe ear. Not the most glamorous part one can play in another person's life, but an important one.

MAKE CHRISTMAS WITH WHAT YOU'VE GOT

We were in production for *Chitty Chitty Bang Bang* for almost a year in Europe; we shot everywhere from a studio in London to the French countryside to Bavaria. It was far from the smooth, joyous shoot that *Mary Poppins* had been: long weather delays, the aforementioned child-hating director, the constant push to make the whole movie more and more over-the-top. Producer Albert "Cubby" Broccoli was determined to turn Ian Fleming's humble family adventure novel into a kids' version of James Bond, his wildly popular spy franchise—replete with flashy gizmos, elaborate special effects, and epic locations.

We all struggled through it. Heather Ripley, the girl who played my daughter, was terribly homesick, lonely, and depressed, and no one (including me) picked up on it or stepped in to help. I hobbled through the early weeks of production with a torn calf muscle, and for the rest of the shoot, I was racked with anxiety over what the doctor who treated my injury had told me: I had arthritis, all over my body.

For many months, I was fortunate enough to have my family with me, and I stole away from set whenever I could to be with them. All the while, though, my wife Margie was grappling with inexplicable fatigue and ever-worsening pelvic pain. We tried to tamp down worries and enjoy our fleeting family time, but the strained fun came to an abrupt end when a doctor suggested that Margie might have cervical cancer.

I immediately flew her home with the kids for testing and then flew home briefly myself to help her through. Thank God she didn't have cancer, but flying back to Europe alone to finish the movie was agony, then finding out Cubby (who had urged me to go home) had docked my pay for my absence just soured me on the whole project.

Luckily, I still have my son Barry around to help me recall one of the most magical bright spots in that whole gloom-clouded experience.

While shooting in England, my family rented a beautiful old red house outside London. It felt kind of creepy and haunted, very on-brand for the Halloween-obsessed Van Dykes. The third floor was particularly mysterious. It had a huge working fireplace in the living room that kept the place at least a little warm.

We were there for Christmas. But with none of the ornaments, lights or tinsel from back home in California, we decided to take matters into our own hands.

Behind the house was a little bit of woods, and I took the whole family back there to find a tree. We made our choice, I sawed it down, and we dragged it back to the house together, the kids putting in extra muscle to spare my tender calf. I rigged the tree to stand straight-ish and did some trimming to make it look triangular-ish, then we all spent hours poking needles through popped popcorn and cranberries and stringing them together. When we draped the strings over the branches, that tree looked spectacular.

Reliving that day with Barry now, we both feel a little proud of ourselves. Despite the trying circumstances, we were all determined to make our holiday with what we had—which is why it felt so special. Who needs a flying car that turns into a speedboat, a dirigible, naval battles, or air battles or a Vulgarian castle? We had our old-timey homemade Christmas tree.

I'm so lucky to have my sharp-minded son around to help me rediscover joyful forgotten memories like this one. I strongly recommend that everyone equip yourself with a Barry, as soon as you possibly can.

DON'T TRUST MACHINES

Caractacus Potts, my character in *Chitty Chitty Bang Bang*, was a scatterbrained inventor. And his wonky contraptions are what many people remember most fondly about the movie. The carpet cleaner that sucks up the whole carpet; the bike-powered haircutter that renders a man half bald.

Behind the scenes, some of Caractacus's inventions were just as comically unreliable in real life.

The eponymous car was probably the least troublesome. It was a big heavy thing, like a truck, and very hard to steer. Plus, it only had a four-cylinder Ford engine in it, so you couldn't really get it going.

Then there was the amazing Breakfast Machine in the "You Two" song scene. I'm singing with my two kids as I make breakfast using this huge Rube Goldberg–style thing that cracks eggs and plates them with sausage, cooks them up, and delivers them via conveyor belt right to the breakfast table. The Breakfast Machine, along with many other inventions in the movie, was created for the film by Rowland Emmett, a brilliant craftsman of kinetic sculptures.

We three actors adored the Breakfast Machine, but it wasn't always an easy scene partner. Sometimes during filming, it hurled eggs willy-nilly or dropped plates, and the crew had to step in to repair it. We'd be at the table, singing and waiting for the plates to come gliding down in front of us, and the Breakfast Machine would miss its cue. The plates just wouldn't arrive. This meant lots and lots of takes.

The most dangerous invention comes right at the beginning of the movie, Caractacus's Rocket Suit, which is just what it sounds like: a suit made of live fiery rockets, strapped to my back, that are supposed to make me fly. In the scene, the rockets come briefly to life as I try to launch off a wooden ramp, then fizzle out. Then, suddenly, they pop into action again, sending me hurtling back down the ramp, hopping and yelping around the farmyard and through a clothesline, smoking and sparking. Caractacus's kids are cracking up the whole time, and so is the audience.

After we filmed thc scene, I went back to my dressing room and took off my boots to discover that I was completely barefoot. My nylon socks were just gone! They'd been burned off by the rockets! And I hadn't felt a thing.

RECONSIDER THE BOOGEYMAN

Mention *Chitty Chitty Bang Bang* to anyone who first saw the film as a child, and once they've sung a lyric or two of the title song and recalled the Breakfast Machine, their faces will suddenly darken with a long-buried memory come to life again. I have witnessed this phenomenon more times than I can count. They are remembering the film's villain, the Child Catcher.

Wearing a black top hat and coat, sometimes flimsily hidden with the colorful garb of a candy seller, the Child Catcher has a knack for creepy skulking and scampering, and he literally wields a net on a pole to do the deed he's named for.

In his most terrifying scene, the Child Catcher lures little Jemima and Jeremy into the back of his colorful candy wagon, yanks a lever and the coach's cheerful disguise falls away, revealing the children to be trapped in an actual cage. The Child Catcher hops in front, whips the horses into a gallop, and off goes the stagecoach with the kids in back, screaming for their lives.

After filming wrapped and the movie was released, I am embarrassed to admit that it took me a while to really see the

Child Catcher from a kid's point of view. He was the embodiment of the sly predator their parents had taught them to fear. He was the boogeyman! And with the film's regular rerelease in years to follow, he has burrowed himself into the collective unconscious of multiple generations.

Let me now attempt to undo some of the trauma.

The reason that the terror of the Child Catcher didn't dawn on me until later was because I knew the actor who played him, and he was about as far from the boogeyman as you can get. On set, Robert Helpmann was a kind, gentle man. He was unfailingly protective of the child actors, standing up to the director when he cursed in their earshot, always smiling and laughing with them off camera. During filming, they really had to work to act scared of him!

But that's not all there is to know about Helpmann. Next time you dare watch the Child Catcher's scenes, watch his legs and feet. He's not walking across those Bavarian cobblestones; he's prancing and skipping with the precise turnout of a ballet dancer.

Because that's exactly what Helpmann was, an internationally renowned dancer, choreographer, actor, and director. He had danced alongside Moira Shearer in the centerpiece ballet of the 1948 classic film *The Red Shoes,* and when we shot *Chitty Chitty Bang Bang*, he was codirector of the Australian Ballet.

There's another moment of Helpmann's balletic poise that only I and the cast and crew got to witness.

During a rehearsal for one of those stagecoach-driving scenes, Helpmann was sitting up front, coming around a corner when the coach behind him tipped, bringing the whole rig—with Helpmann in it—over with it. Looking on in horror, we all thought he was done for!

But before the stagecoach went fully over, Helpmann managed to swivel out of his seat, step onto the front wagon wheel, and escape. Just as the coach crashed into pieces behind him, he landed safely on the street. It was the most fantastically graceful thing I'd ever seen in my life, like a petit jeté! And keep in mind, Helpmann was well into his fifties at the time!

Then, the finale: with an eye toward us awestruck onlookers, he raised his arms to either side, perfectly poised—half curtsy, half ta-da!

Hopefully, that delightful little performance will, if not erase, then at least balance out some of your festering Child Catcher terror.

TELL YOUR HARDEST STORIES

In December 1973, I found a seat in a circle of chairs in a grim, fluorescent-lit meeting room at the Brentwood Veterans' Hospital. Around me were military vets, young and old, all hospitalized for drug and alcohol addiction and gathered for regular group therapy. I was there as a visitor, doing research for my role as an alcoholic in *The Morning After*, a TV movie being shot elsewhere in the facility.

It was weird for these guys to have a Hollywood actor eavesdropping on their raw, real-life stories of struggle, I could tell. Right off the bat, I needed to assure them that I would be a sympathetic listener. "The subject of the movie is very personal to me," I began, "because I myself am an alcoholic."

Their faces flickered with surprise. At the time, only my family and a handful of other people in my life knew about my drinking problem.

"So, I understand some of what you're going through. But really, I'm here to listen and learn."

With the ice broken, at least a bit, the men were ready to share their stories. Virtually every one of them was harrowing. Many had been drinking or using drugs to self-medicate for war-related trauma and physical injuries. They'd lost children, wives, jobs, and homes to addiction. They'd been violent, suicidal, incarcerated, repeatedly hospitalized. The disease had ravaged their organs and broken their souls.

Once each of them got started, it was hard for them to stop. There was urgency in their storytelling, as if by confessing all the gory details, they might free themselves of some pain. And judging by how their bodies slackened once they'd finished speaking, that seemed to be true.

The other thing that struck me was how they all listened to one another. No matter if their drug was booze or heroin, they nodded along, feeling the parallels in their own stories, shaking their heads at the really bad stuff that hit home too. If something they heard sounded like denial or deflecting responsibility, they'd say so—not to shame the speaker, but to push them to be more honest. They were all in this together, like a brotherhood.

While I was there to only observe, I felt right in there with them, the pain in their stories calling up my own. During my treatment for alcoholism out in Arizona two years earlier, group therapy had been something like this too. But after rehab, I'd been eager to put that experience behind me. I was "fixed," I had told myself, done with all this "healing through sharing" stuff. Now, it was reawakening, uncomfortably, inside me: not just how powerful this tool of sharing was, but how much I'd neglected it.

Finally, in the silence I thought signified the meeting was winding down, an older guy turned to me and said: "So, Mr. Van Dyke. What's *your* story?"

My whole body went tense.

I barely touched alcohol until my late twenties, at which point I became the stereotypical drinker to a T. Like millions of Americans in the late 1950s, I was starting a new life with my family in the suburbs, where dinner parties were how you made friends with your neighbors. Cocktails were all but essential for pushing through social anxiety and having some fun. More new friends meant more dinner parties and more cocktails, and soon, everybody—including me—was downing a fourth martini before the flambé.

By the mid-'60s, we'd moved from suburban Long Island to Los Angeles and my movie and TV career was booming. Now, the bourbon started flowing as soon as I left work, and continued at home, unabated until bedtime. My wife Margie was drinking too, always right there to snatch the bottle before I put it down. It was our go-to way to relax.

By 1967, there were whispers at work—not that I was drinking on the job (I wasn't), but I was always kvetching about my hangovers. I heard this from a friend, who gently suggested I might want to seek help, to which—again, true to stereotype—I sputtered out a bunch of defensive *thank you, but I'm fine*s and forgot all about it. And there were always other "real" drunks I could point out to assure myself that I was indeed fine: the slurrers and stumblers at parties, the three-martini lunchers from work, all those perpetually hammered movie stars.

A year or so later, Margie's long-simmering unhappiness with our life in Los Angeles came to a head, and she insisted that the family move full-time to our ranch in Arizona. She relished the desert solitude, and I couldn't stand it. My nights got boozier and boozier.

One hungover morning in 1972, I sat in our kitchen studying my shaking hands and allowed myself to see a pattern: I had been fighting with Margie much more often, and losing my temper with our four kids more too. And all my barking and snarling only really happened at night. My extended "happy hour" had become anything but.

I was pushing my wife to tears. I was scaring my kids. I was doing real emotional damage to my family. And when I finally accepted that, I felt horrified and so ashamed.

Right away, I couldn't live with being that person a second longer. I jumped into husbandly-fatherly fix-it mode, drove down to the local hospital and checked myself in for a three-week treatment plan. This is my naturally impatient way, but there's another thing too: other than telling my wife and kids that I was seeking help for my drinking before I left, I wasn't ready to process how it had affected our family. I needed to do this part alone.

Once in treatment, I again tried to deny I *really* had a problem, garnering a chorus of *oh, please*s from the counselors and my fellow patients in group therapy. By the end of my three weeks, I was able to admit I was an alcoholic, but I also thought now the hard part was over. As soon as I was out, Margie went in herself for own addiction, to antianxiety medication, which was obviously intertwined with mine.

Back at home together, we talked it through with our kids, tearfully apologizing for what we'd put them through and explaining what we knew about our addictions. Yes, they were relieved and forgiving. But I'm also pretty sure they had their doubts that Mom and Dad were really "all better now."

Indeed, we weren't. We were at the starting point of the protracted dissolution of our marriage. More immediately, I moved back to LA alone and promptly relapsed—only long enough to down four bourbons, but I felt so sick and humiliated, like I was back at square one.

Not long after, in an amazingly fortuitous twist, the script for *The Morning After* came my way—a brutal drama about a successful PR writer whose drinking shatters his family and destroys his life. This was groundbreaking territory. In the early 1970s, nobody wanted to talk about alcoholism. It was a source of private shame (as I knew firsthand) and so much dangerous misunderstanding.

For me, the movie seemed to be fate. My drinking problem felt like a failure, and now, here was a way to give it a greater purpose. I knew I could help so many people with this movie, if we did it right. Also, subconsciously, I hoped that giving my creative life over to the issue of alcoholism would help me stay focused on my sobriety.

First, I confessed my own alcoholism to my agents, then the movie's director, then my costars—all of whom were surprised, but overwhelmingly supportive. And very discreet with what was still my dirty little secret.

Which brings me up to my December 1973 research visit at the veterans' hospital where we were shooting. In that meeting, I did end up sharing my story with those other addicts, as prompted. It was more of a hurried summary, to be honest, and part of me felt embarrassed by how tame and privileged my experiences were compared to theirs. The funny thing is they didn't feel that way at all. They were right there with me, just as I had been with them. At its root, our disease was the same.

After the meeting, I thanked the hospital staff and all the vets for sharing their stories. Their honesty had moved me deeply, and I vowed to bring that honesty to my performance and the movie as a whole.

As I walked across the hospital campus to the wing where filming would soon begin, an uneasy feeling washed over me. I'd said the *film* would be honest. My *performance* as an alcoholic.

Then, it hit me like a ton of bricks. Was I really going to do this movie, meant to destigmatize and open a conversation about alcoholism, all the while keeping my own alcoholism a secret?!

What was I thinking?! That, somehow if I could make a difference with my acting, that would let me off the hook from having to talk about my actual struggle as a person? Wouldn't that be hypocritical? Wouldn't that be hiding?!

Man, I was so deep in the screwed-up thinking that comes with this disease—shame, denial, abdication of responsibility. I wasn't fixed at all!

"No, no, the shoot's going great," I reassured my startled agents from the hospital pay phone a few hours later. "But I'm thinking it makes sense for me to, I mean given the subject matter, to go public about, you know, my own drinking problem."

A long silence ensued, in which I pictured my agents' heads exploding in unison.

Finally, one of them mustered up a shaky question: "You mean . . . when we're doing press before the movie airs?"

"No actually, I was thinking right now. I really want to do it right now."

Another long silence. "Dick. No."

Then they got into their reasons. Predictably, they were worried about my image and bankability. *Playing* an alcoholic was one thing; *being* an alcoholic in real life was a whole other ballgame.

But that's exactly the problem, I retorted. This stigma is keeping everybody in hiding. Which means they're not getting help! Which means many of them are dying!

My agents could hear in my voice that I'd already made the decision. Still, they begged me to sleep on it.

Reader, I did not.

I hung up and called a reporter who I knew and trusted. The next morning, she came over to the hospital, and during a break from filming I sat down with her, in the flimsy hospital gown I was wearing for the scene—my character had just been committed to the psych ward. Which was pretty much how I felt at that moment with my alcoholism, raw and flailing, two years into recovery and still deep in its toxic psychology.

Mindful of just how much I had been lying to myself, I committed to giving the reporter the whole truth. I told her everything I've just told you, every step of my journey as a problem drinker, all the intertwined life circumstances, my transformation "from happy drunk to hostile and aggressive," rehab, relapse, the confusion and self-deception that persisted still. "I must admit," I said to her, when it comes to pinpointing why I became an alcoholic, "I'm still sorting out the real reasons from the alibis."

The story got picked up across the country. As expected, when Mr. Goody Two-shoes admitted his addiction to the world, the public was shocked. Friends and colleagues from wherever I'd lived and worked called to offer sympathy and encouragement, reporting that they, and everyone they knew, could barely believe the news. Within a week, I was getting letters by the thousand—people were moved and incredibly understanding, many detailing how alcoholism had impacted them and their loved ones too.

That reaction spurred me to go even more public. I appeared on *The Dick Cavett Show*, one of the best interviews I've ever done, and I told my story onstage in Washington, DC, for a press conference with other celebrity alcoholics. I am told that rehab facilities still show *The Morning After* to this day.

The movie came out beautifully, to wide critical acclaim. I even got an Emmy nomination! As proud as I am of the whole thing, it's the final scenes that really stand out. Having snuck out of a psych ward, my character beelines to a bar, downs a stiff drink and calls his wife to say that he's lost the battle. In the next scene, he has spiraled much further, bearded and disheveled, stumbling through a highway underpass with a bottle in a bag. At the end of the tunnel, he's at the beach. He sits down to drink and watch the sunset and seagulls, in utter defeat.

I'd had to fight for that ending. The network wanted the movie to wrap up happily, with rehab and my character getting well. On this point, I had been adamant. A happy ending would let people with drinking problems think: *Well, I can get to this recovery thing eventually and it will all work out.* In fact, if you don't get help and stick with it, alcoholism will kill you.

There is an important point to why I am telling you this story—about telling my story. Because it has saved my life.

It took many iterations—from what I said in my own rehab to the veterans' group to the reporter to Dick Cavett, to my family and my therapist—for me to get increasingly honest with myself: to admit my relapses, to see clearly how my drinking had impacted my relationships and my sense of self, to really understand alcoholism as a disease. Far more than the act of quitting itself, that ongoing process of deepening my story was the thing that really healed me.

Each time I put a new layer of it into words, I felt a release of the power that alcoholism had over me. I was separating myself from the disease, seeing my experience as a battle with the disease. Telling my story was giving *me* power and freedom.

Each of us has our own hard stories of crisis and struggle. When we hold them in, out of fear or shame, they control us. But when we tell our stories, we're in the driver's seat. And when we share those stories, even just among our friends and family, we are literally helping one another to survive, just like that brotherhood of vets.

PLAY AGAINST TYPE

The Morning After wasn't the only role where I ran screaming from the "Dick Van Dyke persona"—the goofs, the physical comedy, the affability, all of it. In the 1970s, my whole life was unraveling, and I was not at all a funny, carefree person. I felt just like the Great Malaise itself: smoggy and glum.

As successful as I had been channeling my own experiences into *The Morning After*, I had a bit more trouble with the darker stuff a few years later. In the period drama *The Runner Stumbles,* I played a priest whose faith is challenged by his secret affair with a nun.

Emotionally speaking, there was some heavy overlap with my life at the time. I'd been having a relationship (with my future partner Michelle), and my marriage to Margie had decisively fallen apart. And, having given up organized religion some years before, I was still struggling with faith and spirituality.

Somehow though, I didn't feel ready for the part of the priest. Maybe my own midlife upheaval was just too close and unresolved for me to use it as an actor. Maybe I was relying, instead, on an intellectual understanding of the character.

Whatever was going on, I felt lost for the entire shoot. The title of the movie was like an in-joke on me.

As if sensing my discomfort, my beloved director Stanley Kramer would overdo it on his praise for my good scenes, slamming his fist into my shoulder and yelling: "Good job, buddy!" It got to be where I flinched whenever he came near me.

I haven't had the courage to rewatch this movie in forever, so I don't know how my performance stands up. I think I can live with "Good job, buddy!"

Looking back, I'm glad I stretched myself as an actor, even when I struggled. I was really trying to grow, to tap into new parts of who I am through those roles. Going out of your comfort zone, doing something that is unfamiliar or uncomfortable, is the only way you can hope to change.

Sometimes during that period, I went way out of my comfort zone, daring to play the coldhearted villain—if only briefly—as a guest star on a single episode of TV. I now present the incomplete works of Dark Van Dyke.

In the mystery series *Columbo,* I played the slimiest, most unlikable villain you can imagine: a man who so loathes his (admittedly abrasive) wife that he ties her up and kills her, then to cover it up, frames a guy for her kidnapping and kills him too. I gave that cold evil my all.

At the same time, I brought out the comedy in the show's star, Peter Falk, famously known for his glass eye. Rehearsing one scene, I knocked on the door, and he opened it with a wad of tissue in his empty eye socket. I lost it.

This episode came back to me in vivid detail only very recently, when I received a rather odd autograph request in the mail: a photo of me as that villain, holding the rope.

In NBC's infamously expensive flop series *Supertrain*, I guest starred as (what the audience thinks is) a psychopathic hit man. In one scene, I'm carrying a glass of (possibly poisoned) milk down the train corridor to my victim's suite, shot from below to make me, and the milk, look as ominous as possible.

But then there's a preposterous twist ending which undermines all my good work as a bad guy! The milk wasn't poisoned at all; I was actually a secret good Samaritan! Come on!

Years later, as a guest star on my son Barry's show *Airwolf*, I went full supervillain. My character was Malduke (!) a rich, powerful, and unblinking madman with a very convoluted mission involving threats to blow up a barge carrying toxic waste. In Malduke's lair, his minions regularly administered infusions of some mysterious serum into my arm.

The climax was the most fun. I get to choke Barry in a fight, then I'm thrown into a wall of circuitry, which sends me into a paroxysm of smoke and sparks. Then my head pops off and rolls onto the floor, revealing me to be a robot. For the "head shot," I stood in a hole cut out of the set's floor and gave my best dead robot stare.

I never really believe myself as an evil villain, but apparently some people did. I've heard anecdotally that, when some younger viewers saw cheerful Bert show up as a killer in *Columbo*, it shattered their innocence.

I suppose these archvillain guest spots were a little like the military for me back when I was seventeen: they showed me who I wasn't. I'm grateful for my amusing detour into darkness, but I am so glad I didn't get lost there.

RETIRE ON YOUR OWN TERMS

In 1993, Andy Griffith warned me not to sign up for *Diagnosis: Murder*. He made a great case too. At the time, I was sixty-eight, which a lot of people consider retirement age. Andy was about that age, too, and having spent the prior seven years helming his own "geriatric mystery" show, *Matlock*, he knew well the toll an hour-long drama can take on an older fellow.

"I cannot tell you how hard it is," he said.

We hung up and I thought it over. When easygoing Andy Griffith says "hard" fifty times in a five-minute chat, you better listen.

The thing is, I didn't feel ready to retire. It felt like giving up my identity, my passion, my whole purpose in life. It felt like defeat.

On the other hand, I knew, if I put my mind to it, I could probably map out a vision for retirement that was plenty fulfilling, with less "hard" ways to keep performing. A play or something. But figuring that out felt hard too!

By that time, CBS had been kind of nudging me into the show, bit by bit. I started in the part of Mark Sloan, eccentric crime-solving physician as a guest star on another TV show, *Jake and the Fatman*, then they spun my character out into a TV movie. Then another. Then another.

In the producers' minds, it was all but inevitable that I'd carry on with the role in a series. Just for one season, they told me.

Finally, I convinced myself that I believed them.

Hah!

Renewal after renewal after renewal followed. *Diagnosis: Murder* continued for eight full seasons—something like 180 hour-long episodes! Andy beat me by a season with *Matlock*, but Angela Lansbury trounced us both with twelve seasons of *Murder, She Wrote*. Not that we still felt competitive at our age or anything.

The point is: eight seasons and I survived!

How did I do it? What was my secret?

Well, basically, instead of actually retiring, I took all the things the AARP tells us to do in our retirement and brought them to work with me. Consequently, I had the time of my life.

First, I prioritized "family time." For the *Diagnosis* TV movies, I brought my son Barry on to play my detective son, and he came along for the series too. Think about that: While I'm working, I also get to hang out with my kid, day in and day out! It was father-son bonding at its finest, a real friendship.

Over the course of the show's run, Barry and I ended up bringing on a whole gaggle of other family members too: my brother, Jerry; my daughter Stacy; my daughter's husband Kevin; and all four of Barry's kids. That's eight Van Dykes (and one McNally) on a single show! How's that for nepotism?

I also stayed fit. One of my favorite of Dr. Mark Sloan's many quirks was his love of on-the-job roller-skating. He's often seen zipping down the hospital halls on wheels, visiting patients and checking charts. No stunt double necessary—I came to the part with skating skills at the ready. For a time, we shot in a real hospital in Denver that had these gorgeous smooth marble floors—I could really get going in there.

Finally, I did all the things I loved. To be specific, here are some of the other pastimes and hobbies that just happened to find their way into the mix of Dr. Mark Sloan's character.

- Dances, especially soft-shoe
- Does magic tricks
- Listens to jazz
- Plays many musical instruments
- Sings in a barbershop quartet

Any of that sound familiar?

I realize I was lucky to "not really retire" on my own terms. A lot of people don't have that choice at all; they have to keep working long after they're ready to stop. But these "rules" can apply to everyone in need of a fulfilling vision for their golden years, whether or not they're still working.

REMAIN ANONYMOUS

One day on *Diagnosis: Murder*, we were shooting in a hotel or something, and while the crew was rigging the lights, they set up chairs for me and my son Barry out on a loading dock that opened right onto the street. Some people would walk or drive by, peek and see me and kind of wave.

But then one guy pulls up, points at me in recognition and bellows: "Dick Van Dyke!"

I smiled politely and said "Yeah, how you doing?"

By way of response, he dropped his index finger and raised his middle one and screamed, "F*** you!" then drove off.

We sat there stunned for a second and then cracked up. We never laughed so hard.

I guess not everybody's a fan.

START A BAND

Old age is a lot like young adulthood, if you play it right. You're free to reinvent yourself, make new friends, take up new hobbies, or even start up a band. Though for *me* in retirement age, starting a band looks a lot different than what a teenager might do.

There is some backstory: In 1980 I starred in a revival of *The Music Man*, which toured across the country, then ran at City Center in New York. Most of my day-to-day attention was devoted to honing my performance as Harold Hill. But there was a foursome of secondary characters that I was always drawn to: the long-feuding members of River City's school board whom Harold Hill coaxes into togetherness . . . by turning them into a barbershop quartet!

What a marvel, how each of their voices melded with the others to create the most soul-tingling harmonies. I wanted so badly to be part of that. And I had the perfect bass for it too.

Before each show, I would ask the bass singer if he was feeling okay, hoping he might admit to having a cold or something, so I could stand in for him. At the beginning of the number "Lida Rose," I leave the stage, and the quartet takes over, eventually including Marian the librarian, who takes the song to the most beautiful place. Every performance, I was hovering in the wings, singing along to the bass.

For twenty years, I quietly nursed my love of that sound. In 1999, I worked some barbershop singing into an episode of *Diagnosis: Murder*, but that was a fleeting fix.

A year later, I got what I'd been hankering for, in the most accidental of ways. Meet Mike Mendyke, Bryan Chadima, and Eric Bradley, the other three founding members of The Vantastix. During breaks in a recent rehearsal, they helped me remember the full story of "How the Band Got Together."

MIKE: I'd only been living in LA for a few weeks, so I was kind of naive when it came to celebrity sightings. I walk into a Starbucks in Malibu and there's Dick, and the first words that popped out of my mouth were: "Oh my God, you're Dick Van Dyke!"

DICK: I said, "Yes, I am."

MIKE: The second thing I said was "I understand you're a big fan of barbershop music."

DICK: Not something you hear every day.

MIKE: I love barbershop. I'd been singing it as a side gig for years.

BRYAN: Mike's day job is rocket scientist.

ERIC: He's not joking.

DICK: Coincidentally, I had been trying to start a barbershop group up at the exact same time. I'd even put an ad in the paper. Nobody answered.

MIKE: Maybe if you'd put your name in it?

DICK: I asked Mike if he had any other guys—

MIKE: And I immediately thought of Bryan and Eric.

DICK: So I invited them all over to sing!

MIKE: I didn't entirely believe it was real until we got there. We all showed up at his house, and I'd say 70 percent of that first meeting, we just sat around listening to Dick tell stories.

ERIC: He kept telling us how he didn't think he was a very good singer and was scared to go onstage and sing by himself.

BRYAN: Which was odd because isn't that what you did your whole life?

DICK: In my defense, a cappella is very different than musical theater. There's no accompanist, so it's all on you.

BRYAN: The whole first visit was very disarming. We were all just pinching ourselves. By the end of it, we realized: Okay, there's no catch here. Dick just wants us to hang out and talk and arrange songs and teach him to sing them. So that's what we started doing.

Becoming The Vantastix meant devoting months of regular rehearsal time to bring our voices together into harmony. Existing barbershop and a cappella arrangements helped, but all of us knew we really wanted to be doing fresh material, unique to us.

So, Bryan undertook the incredible project of creating original arrangements, reworking classics we all adored into four-part vocal scores. Each new arrangement Bryan brought to the table was a gem, as was Mike's reworking of "Chitty Chitty Bang Bang." They translated instrumentals into vocals with such musical wit, which made the challenge of learning the songs a constant joy.

I gravitated toward the snappier numbers because I really like to move when I sing. But there was one ballad, "Baby Mine," the mother elephant's lullaby in *Dumbo*, that always broke our hearts.

MIKE: I used to sing that to my daughter when she was a baby, and so every time we did it as a group, it was hard for me not to cry.

DICK: Remember when we used to rehearse over at your place in Calabasas? And there she was in her little rocker?

MIKE: Yeah, now she can tell people that Dick Van Dyke sang her to sleep when she was a baby.

ERIC: Or kept her awake.

When it came time to take our act public, we started small, doing charity dinners, benefits, and local events.

Our first big Hollywood opportunity was a spot at the Society of Singers' 2001 Ella Award ceremony honoring my old friend and *Mary Poppins* costar Julie Andrews. It took some real work to get that gig. The Vantastix were a bunch of complete unknowns back then, so we had to drive over to the producers' house for an in-person audition. Which we aced.

The guys always like to remind me of an early performance we did for nurses at a hospital in Orange County.

BRYAN: Those nurses were hot to trot for you, Dick.

ERIC: We had to sneak you out back because they were rushing the stage!

This story always gives me a kick. Like it's 1964 and the nurses are American teenage girls, and we're The Beatles.

The next decade was up, up, up for The Vantastix. At Pepperdine University, we sang "Lida Rose" for Shirley Jones herself, who'd sung that song in the film version of *The Music Man*. We had a national television appearance on Nick at Night's *TV Land*. We sung at the Hollywood Bowl, a venue so gigantic that it gave me stage fright. And in 2010, we performed at an Independence Day concert at Ford's Theater in Washington, with President Barack Obama and First Lady Michelle Obama bobbing along in the front row.

The Barbershop Invasion was real. The Vantastix had arrived!

MIKE: At first, we kind of thought this will be fun for a few years and then Dick will get bored of us, or get old or something, and that'll be that. Twenty-five years later, we're still here.

DICK: And you guys are still not even as old as I was when we first got together!

MIKE: We're catching up, Dick. Don't worry.

DICK: I'll wait.

COMMIT TO PLAY

Playing came naturally to all of us as kids. Then, somewhere along the way, some of us decided we had more serious and important things to do with ourselves and so we gave up play.

Luckily for me, I got to keep playing through my entire career. As seriously as I took it, comedy, singing and dancing were always just my way to feel and express simple pure joy. To this day, I hum through my whole daily routine, I crack jokes and pull pranks, and I make my body go rubbery—just for the fun of it.

This has kept me connected not just with the child inside me, but the children in my family and all the children I encounter out in the world. Nothing beats playing with a kid, even for just a moment. It frees you both in a miraculous way.

But the thing is: you have to really let go and go for it. And you can't possess a selfish, ulterior motive. Case in point:

Filming *Mary Poppins*, nearly every on- and off-camera moment with my enthusiastic young costars, seven-year-old Matthew Garber and eight-year-old Karen Dotrice, felt like playtime. Our ceiling tea party number "I Love to Laugh" required us all to be suspended high in the air by wires for days on end, and it never got old. Sure, acrophobic Matthew had to be bribed a dime for each time he was lifted, but once we were all up there, we giggled and spun in our comfy plaster-cast "butt seats" like we were on a magic swing set.

During all our time waiting around between takes, I did every ridiculous stumble and exaggerated injury I could think of to keep things lively. For me and the kids, this was a fully mutual game: their laughter brought me energy and enthusiasm.

Even when fidgety Matthew took to biting my leg out of boredom, I felt his weird little nips as a form of affection. Maybe he was playing with a loose tooth?

When the mirth felt forced, however, Matthew would not play along. Filming solo close-ups, the director wanted Matthew to laugh on command right to the camera, but with nothing to actually find funny, he wasn't feeling it at all. He wouldn't even crack a smile, no matter what anyone tried.

So, they enlisted child-at-heart me to stand behind the camera and tickle Matthew's funny bone. I made every silly face I could think of, and I even pulled out a slew of fresh pratfalls. No luck. Matthew simply refused to laugh.

As humbling as that was for me, I really got it. As Matthew could see, there was purpose and pressure in all my comic contortions. I wasn't just playing.

If you want to play with a child, you've got to be honest in your intentions.

And of course, it's much easier when they've got a head start on you.

In 2021, I received a Kennedy Center Award. The event was packed with incredibly talented adults, from my fellow honorees Debbie Allen, Joan Baez, and Garth Brooks to Chita Rivera and Dr. Anthony Fauci. Amid the crowd backstage, I spotted a one-year-old girl bobbing along to the background music, and I stopped in my tracks. She was exuberantly lost in her little moves, radiating spirit.

When you see somebody dancing like that, it sparks something primal. It sucks you right in. Suddenly, I wanted nothing to do with small talk or any talk at all. I wanted to dance too!

So, I launched into my best rendition of her moves. She looked up at me, immediately got what was happening, and bounced right back at me.

We were off to the races! We were dancing together! Trading moves, back and forth, ear-to-ear grins and no words necessary. I was awestruck at how present and focused we were together, and I never wanted our dance to end.

As it turns out, she was Debbie Allen's granddaughter, so of course movement was in her blood! For me, that toddler was the eccentric stranger you meet at a stiff wedding and stay glued to all night. Long after I forget the rest of the event, I will still feel electrified by the connection we danced our way into.

Playing with kids like that is one of the big reasons I still feel so young. Emotionally, it has kind of a table-clearing effect: all the stuff I might be unhappy about or ruminating over just ceases to matter. It ceases to *exist*! In playtime, life feels weightless.

To see what I mean, seek out a lesson from the pros, our Elders of Play. This requires, at first, proving yourself as a worthy student.

Next time you encounter a little kid, crying or looking glum, make a funny face at them. But do so with pure intentions, not because you're annoyed with them or they're making noise, but because you genuinely want to see them happy.

Don't worry if your first try fails to elicit even a tiny smirk. Any self-respecting child is not just going to drop their whole hard-earned foul mood for one lazy gesture of adult silliness.

Now, if you've got a repertoire of ridiculous expressions to show off, that tells them you might, in fact, be the real deal: somebody who's truly committed to getting foolish. A kid in grown-up disguise who's ready to play.

If you've really given it your all, chances are the kid won't just be laughing, they'll be trading crazy expressions back and forth with you until your face hurts.

Connecting with children through body movement works the same way. And it doesn't have to start with outright dancing either. Maybe a kid is twirling their hair or just fidgeting.

Twirl and fidget back at them. Add your own flourishes. Watch their eyes light up when they realize that you are *communicating* with them.

And if you keep the conversation going, it's all but guaranteed that your silent little duet will expand from fingers to arms to legs and, eventually, your whole bodies.

Congratulations! Face your partner and take a bow. And don't be surprised if they ask for an encore.

Long after these little moments of play are over, you can bask in their afterglow. The more you play with kids, the more the spirit of play infuses your adult being, and everything else you're doing in adult life. You can tap into play to make practically anything more fun—a strained family visit, a boring car ride, a dreaded chore, an anxious wait at the doctor's office.

As all these little experiences accumulate, your whole approach to living can change. Your whole self becomes buoyant!

Now, really. Try it out for yourself and see. Go play.

Just play.

SAVE ALL THAT ARTWORK

After the Western matinees on Saturdays, my childhood friends and I couldn't get those movies out of our heads. We'd talk about them all the way home. Then, after we practiced the death-falls we'd seen in our backyard, we'd go inside and sit for hours, drawing out in pencil or pen all the scenes we remembered! The details of the shoot-outs and chases, vocalizing all the bullet noise and stuff and the dialogue as we drew. It was a great way to keep the thrill of the movie alive. Like you're drawing your own rerun!

Also, for me, drawing for hours on end—focusing so intently on all the details of a single thing—had a meditative effect that was just pure pleasure. From then on, it became my lifelong go-to what-to-do-with-your-hands activity. Creatively, it is a welcome relief from performance, but that childhood ritual also hooked me on the social pleasure of drawing. Hanging around at dinners or cocktail parties, or on the set of my TV shows, I was always sketching, doodling, doing caricatures of all the friends around me.

Hands down, "social art making" was most fun with my kids. My son Barry was convinced I could draw anything, so he'd ask me to draw whatever came into his head. One time, he asked me to draw a rhinoceros, his favorite animal, and he sat there giggling in disbelief, watching me just draw it out perfectly.

After that, he became kind of like my director. *What can I get Dad to draw next?*

The other day, Barry described some of our masterpieces that he'd hung on to and I'd forgotten. They were india-ink movie-paintings! Just like I'd made in childhood! All the vivid details Barry remembered, you'd think we'd done them yesterday, not sixty-some years ago.

One was from a Western we must have seen. Barry asked me if I could draw cowboys in a shoot-out. And boy did I ever, apparently. One guy had his gun drawn, the other guy is flying backward, just shot. I even got the whole town in there!

With another one, we must have just seen a movie with fighter planes. I did an elaborate dogfight, with a Fokker and a SPAD, machine guns blazing and everything. Barry said it was astonishing.

It was just such a pleasure sitting with my son as he remembered and described these pictures. I could kind of see him again as a little boy.

Maybe one of these days, Barry will find those drawings buried in his attic and show them to his grandkids. Or maybe they're long gone. Either way, he has the memory of them, and now so do I.

They are our shared artifacts. And just like a sacred relic dug up at an archaeological dig, they're about so much more than the thing itself. They're about the human ritual surrounding it. Barry and Dad, making our movies together.

BELIEVE IN FATE

We all have a few major turning points in our lives where, looking back later, the difference between "before" and "after" is crystal clear. It wasn't just one part of life that changed. It was everything.

On January 28, 2007, I was eighty-one—for many people, an age where the only big turning point ahead is full-body expiration. For me, though, that day was a much brighter turning point, one that showed me a future where death didn't belong. It was the day I met Arlene.

In February 2025, she and I celebrated our thirteenth wedding anniversary, and as we are often inclined to do, we marveled together at how that momentous day unfolded. It's important for you to hear this story from both horses' mouths, since this day changed Arlene's life as much as it did mine.

Everybody who's married has these coming-together stories, and in their telling and retelling, the role of pedestrian happenstance tends to get turned into "the hand of fate." Arlene and I are no different.

Except in our case, it's really true.

ARLENE: The story actually starts a few days before we met.

I was going to lunch with some friends in Hollywood,

where I was working at a makeup school. First, I remember walking right by your star on the sidewalk, and then my friends got all excited and pointed over to the El Capitan Theatre, where *Mary Poppins* was playing. I had never seen it and they were appalled.

DICK: Criminal.

ARLENE: Then three days later, I was doing makeup at the Screen Actors Guild Awards, and, I didn't know this at the time, you were there to introduce Julie Andrews for her Lifetime Achievement Award. It can be hard working on those shows—they keep a very tight leash on where you can and can't go backstage, so I'm always just moving around, trying to find a spot where I won't get in trouble. Somebody suggested I go into the green room to watch the show on the monitors, so I went in there—

DICK: I saw you as soon as you walked in. And I just felt drawn to you.

ARLENE: You were talking to Cate Blanchett.

DICK: Is that who it was?

ARLENE: And then there was Anthony Hopkins. The whole room was movie stars.

DICK: You walked by me, and I don't know what came over me. Without even thinking, I said: "Hi, I'm Dick."

ARLENE: I knew he was Dick Van Dyke. The first thing I remembered was "Stop, drop, and roll!"—those fire safety ads you were in in the 1970s. When I was in grade school.

DICK: I had never approached a strange woman in my life—that kind of thing terrified me. So how I ever got up the nerve to approach you, I'll never know.

ARLENE: Besides those ads, I didn't know his movies. At the time, the only musicals I really knew were *Grease* and *Sound of Music*.

DICK: I think she thought I was Christopher Plummer.

ARLENE: No, stop!

DICK: You thought I was Christopher Plummer.

ARLENE: That's not true. I'd never seen any of his movies, but I remembered the marquee from the movie theater and, finally, that kind of clicked a little. So I said: "Weren't you in *Mary Poppins*?"

DICK (laughing): That's not something I get every day. Suddenly, all the other backstage chitchat just wasn't interesting anymore.

ARLENE: We talked for a little bit, then he sat us down with the whole cast of *The Mary Tyler Moore Show* and introduced me to Valerie Harper. "This is Arlene Silver," like I was his best friend or something!

DICK: We just talked and talked.

ARLENE: Then, he asked for a card because he said he wanted to put me up for a makeup job on a Hallmark movie he was about to do—

DICK: Something inside me was just screaming: Don't let this person go.

ARLENE: I didn't get any of that. I just thought: Wow, he seems really nice. Maybe a new friend! I gave him my very last card.

DICK: I'm sure I still have it.

ARLENE: It's crazy to think: the chances of us meeting were zero. We were never in the same worlds in entertainment. I was never out in Malibu. You would never come to Silverlake.

DICK: It makes you believe in fate.

ARLENE: So, the very next day, I got this email that totally looked like spam.

Subject: you

Arlene,

I'm afraid I was so smitten with you last night I couldn't think of anything to say.

Still, when the project at Hallmark starts, I'd like to give you a chance to talk with them. Would that be okay?

Dick Van Dyke

ARLENE: I thought, what's with this "smitten"? Is he coming on to me? That hadn't even occurred to me when we were talking! And it turns out, he had a partner, Michelle, and they had been together happily for thirty years.

DICK: Maybe smitten was too strong a word. But it felt right when I wrote it.

Stay tuned: there's more to come in the story of our friendship and eventual romance. But what's important about this particular moment—our first meeting—is that, for both of us, it felt like destiny. Arlene had literally been given two signs in a row a few days before. And for me, it was like some unexplainable force propelling me to talk to her.

This kind of thing had rarely happened to either of us before, if ever. And what's amazing is that we both paid attention! Fate gave us a completely mysterious invitation, and we both RSVP'd in the affirmative!

TAKE YOUR DOUBTS TO THE DESERT

So, I may have overdone it with the "smitten" email to Arlene. My long-term partner Michelle and I were as bonded as two souls can be. I wasn't trying to seduce Arlene or anything. I just wanted to be around her.

Meanwhile, when Arlene went up for the Hallmark job doing my makeup, she was juggling all kinds of conflicting signals, unbeknownst to oblivious me.

ARLENE: I called Stacy Halax, Dick's makeup person from *Diagnosis: Murder* for some tips, and right away, he sounded like a nightmare. "He doesn't like to sit in the chair too long. He needs eye drops. Don't talk to him. Everybody talks to him. And he likes airbrush—do you do airbrush?"

Luckily, I worked at a makeup school, and my friend Rochelle who taught there let me borrow her airbrush machine. So, the day before, I'm practicing airbrush makeup on a doll head, thinking Oh my God, white hair, tan makeup. I am in trouble.

DICK: Hah!

ARLENE: My tryout went fine, thank God, Dick wasn't any kind of diva at all, and so I got the job. The first day I'm doing his makeup, though, he's acting kind of weird.

DICK: I would not get up out of that chair.

ARLENE: He melted into the chair.

DICK: Her face just looked so peaceful to me.

ARLENE: So, every morning as I do his makeup, he's telling me all these stories—Mary Tyler Moore, Sophia Loren, Cary Grant—and I can tell he's nervous.

DICK: For days, I just double-talked. Or I couldn't talk at all. I was so afraid I'd say something stupid.

ARLENE: And you never would eat in front of me. You were so nervous!

Eventually, I was able to relax, and over the course of that movie and a few other projects after that, Arlene and I developed a friendship that felt easy and natural for both of us.

Then, in the span of two short years, I lost both the women I'd loved most in the world: Margie, my ex-wife and the mother of our children, and my partner Michelle, who had suffered through terminal cancer at home for a full year.

I was undone. I wandered around the house in a cloud of grief, I barely went outside, I forgot to shower or buy groceries or pay bills. I was a wreck. I'd never been alone like that in my entire life.

Amidst this haze, Arlene came over to offer condolences and have dinner. All my feelings came swirling up together: that sense of deep kinship, the loneliness and flailing, and yes, the "smitten" part. Now, very much the correct word.

For our first date, I tried hard to impress, taking Arlene to dinner at the Magic Castle, a legendary old Hollywood magic club—members-only and I was a charter member. I had not been back since the 1960s, and Arlene had never been there, so it was an adventure for both of us. Unfortunately, there were some complications.

ARLENE: Everybody was just staring at us the whole time, watching us eat. People kept coming up to us and saying hi to Dick, and later they were taking pictures. It was like being out with a unicorn.

DICK: Then the owners come over to talk, and they want to give us the full tour of the place.

ARLENE: The dusty puppet tour.

DICK: We never had a moment to ourselves.

ARLENE: Then at the valet, of course Dick's car is right there, warm and waiting, and he gets in, waves goodbye and zooms off. And I'm just standing there forever, waiting with my ticket.

Our next few dates were much more down-to-earth. I'll be the first to admit it: I was pedal-to-the-metal on our relationship. I was terrified she'd get away! And I can see now that was a lot of pressure.

ARLENE: First of all, there was the celebrity part of it. Going anywhere with you was such a production. The whole world is right up in your face!

DICK: That really freaked you out.

ARLENE: And the age thing. It hadn't been an issue when we were friends, but now, it hit me hard. I couldn't imagine what our life together would be like, with that kind of a difference. Do we have enough in common to do this every day? Can we still do all the fun stuff in life, like travel? What would happen if you started, you know, seeming really old?

DICK: I love you for saying "if" and not "when."

ARLENE: I hadn't thought about that part before!

DICK: I hadn't either. Honestly, I felt so young around you, I just figured like you'd keep me feeling young forever. And you did, so I was right!

ARLENE: You told me "age is just a number" a million times, I remember, but it didn't really sink in.

DICK: Then you had your . . .

ARLENE: I went to Burning Man. I don't know why.

(Reader, if you don't know what Burning Man is, here's what I've gathered: big happening, middle of the desert, camping, music, and the burning of some kind of big wooden man.)

ARLENE: My friends Scott and Kymber, who built the Burning Man city, basically kidnapped me and took me out there to their camp. I am not a camper. I was covered in sand for three days and all I wanted to do was go home.

DICK: I think you put yourself in that situation on purpose.

ARLENE: I mean it's Burning Man, so it gets kind of existential. I'm sitting around in the desert, out of my comfort zone, so I just kind of opened my mind and started thinking about my life, in a bigger picture way. What did I want to change? What did I want my life to be?

Of course, Dick was very much in the mix of my thinking. When I focused on what our life was, right then, I realized: this is the happiest I have ever been, hands down. Why would I let my mind get in the way of that?

So, I finally let myself feel what Dick was saying. What is age, really? When you love somebody the way we love each other, age is just the last thing that matters. It's meaningless! Dick and I were two kindred souls on this magical adventure, and it was only getting started! I finally really felt that, and it changed my life.

DICK: You went from Burning Man to Aging Man.

ACCEPT "RESCUE" WITH GRACE

At the age of eighty-seven, I thought all my youthful bad luck with cars was in the rearview mirror. Then, one sweltering August afternoon in 2013, I was cruising down the 101 freeway in my beloved white Jaguar XK when smoke began wafting out from under the hood.

What the heck?! I screamed to myself. I had literally just picked up the car from the shop for minor repairs and a tune-up. Did they forget to screw something back on?! Or maybe, just my luck, I'd gotten a flat and the tire was smoking.

Peeved, I pulled over to the side of the highway and called AAA to report what I thought to be a nonemergency breakdown. Shortly after hanging up, however, the wafting smoke became more of a billowing. This was definitely not just burning rubber or a little leaky oil.

Still, I did what I do best in these situations: I stayed perfectly calm. Yes, that smoke might eventually lead to open flames, but I had plenty of time to gather my things and exit my vehicle gracefully.

The only catch: my most important "things" were my CDs and they were all over the car—the glovebox, side pockets, under the seats. I cherished my music collection, but I didn't keep it exactly organized, so this retrieval effort was taking some time. It also involved a lot of hunching over the steering wheel and strained reaching.

The whole time, I was barely aware, if at all, that the smoke up front was getting thicker and blacker, that passing cars were slowing down, and that the people inside those cars were gaping in horror and calling 911. You can imagine what they saw: white-haired man hunched over steering wheel of burning car!

At some point, I heard a voice from behind: "Are you okay? Sir, are you okay?"

Oh boy, I thought, *now people are stopping.*

"I'm fine!" I replied, still stubbornly in my search-and-gather mode.

"You gotta get out of there!" the voice cried—with an urgency I didn't feel was warranted.

"I'm fine! I'm just getting my stuff!"

After some more back-and-forth like that, suddenly my door was open, hands were on my shoulders and I was being hoisted up and yanked backward out of the car—really hard! Amid this unwanted extraction, I managed to grab my bag, which now held at least most of my precious CDs.

Once on my feet and released, I turned to face my grabber: a goateed man with an extremely worried look on his face. My irritation softened.

"Your car's on fire!" he exclaimed. "We need to get back!"

I looked up at the hood—indeed, flames were now beginning to flicker amid the smoke. Still, when it came to the question of moving away, there was a huge disconnect between his sense of imminent danger and my unmet inner desire to do one final CD sweep of the car.

Finally, I gave in and walked with him down the freeway, leaving the car behind. Once he was out of rescue mode, it hit him. "Wait," he said. "Are you Dick Van Dyke?"

We chatted politely for a while as a crowd of other concerned citizens gathered, including some off-duty nurses and/or EMTs who asked if I needed medical attention. I didn't, I replied calmly. I was fine.

All the while, the flames gradually engulfed my entire car, at one point erupting into a loud fireball. Even then, I didn't feel lucky to have narrowly escaped death. I felt sad to lose my Jag.

I called Arlene to break the bad news. Then came the paparazzi, then the fire trucks and police, and finally, Arlene to drive me home.

At first, I handled the barrage of media coverage with grace and humor. Arlene and I posted a picture of my charred car on Twitter with the caption: "Used Jag for sale—REAL CHEAP!!"

Then the news started bothering me. Basically, the emerging narrative was this: "Elderly actor trapped in burning car rescued by stranger seconds before it explodes." My "rescuer" went on CNN to tell his story and was lauded as a "good Samaritan hero," with me falsely cast as the doddering, disoriented victim.

After much eye rolling, I finally let my pride and temper get the better of me and took to Twitter again, to correct the record: "My 'rescue' was like the Boy Scout who helped the old lady across the street, who didn't want to cross the street!!"

In the moment, it felt great to push back, wrest control of the narrative and stick up for my version of events. But almost immediately, I felt a tinge of regret.

It turns out that my good Samaritan had been so consumed with panic I would helplessly die that he swerved off the highway and drove the wrong way up an exit ramp to come back and save me. And, as I learned, he had a reason for taking such urgent action: three weeks earlier, his own wife had been saved by a stranger after a terrible hit-and-run motorcycle crash. "It was just really my husband's turn to be a hero and you know, to really pass that on to someone else," she told one news outlet. "It really moves me a lot."

Well, I'm officially sorry I fired off that curt message. And I'm now able to learn gracefully from my mistake.

While my story was fiery and extreme, it's no different than a more ordinary dilemma we elderly citizens face every day. Strangers are always coming to the rescue when they think we need help, whether it's opening doors, lifting luggage, or swooping in to prevent an imagined fall. Objectively, yes, we should be grateful to be so worried over and looked after.

But it needs to be said that these surprise "rescues" can feel alarming and irritating. Like: "Hey, get out of my space!" Also, sometimes they don't make us feel "cared for," but rather weak and incapable. Especially if we haven't asked for help, and even more especially if we've explicitly told our rescuers, as I did, that "we're fine." These "rescues" call up a feeling that's all too familiar in our golden years: a loss of dignity.

But maybe, I am realizing, there's a less fragile and more authentic dignity to be had here. One that comes from finally being wise enough to see beyond the in-the-moment minutiae of our petty pride and our rescuers' misplaced pity.

It might seem to us older people like there are a surfeit of overeager Boy Scouts in the world. But that's basically the same thing as a baby thinking the whole world is full of people smiling and cooing and wiggling their fingers.

The sad fact is that, for the rest of the population, getting rescued or helped up by a stranger is much more of a rarity. So when it happens to us, whether we asked for it or not, we should celebrate it for what it is: an expression of human kindness, at its most pure.

SEE THE PATTERN TO GET PAST IT

During my CBS years in New York, across the street from the stage door was a cocktail lounge, and I would often stop in for a martini before my commute back to Long Island. The bartender with long red hair was very flirty.

One particular night, she was flirtier than usual. I tried all the standard polite avoidance tricks, but she ignored them all. Finally, I got up to leave and put down my money to pay. She scowled at me and said, loud enough for the whole bar to hear: "What is the matter with you? Don't you like to f***?!"

Everyone in the bar looked up, and I wanted to die. Then, out of my mouth tumbled the ultimate arousal suppressant: "Actually I do . . . but I'm not very good at it."

After that, I never went back there when she was behind the bar.

Unfortunately, this awkward and unwelcome advance was not a one-off. Several years later, on the set of a movie, a barrage of public flirtation from my costar left me rattled for the entire shoot. It happened again with another performer backstage on a TV show. And other times outside of work too. I will spare you the names and details because those aren't what's important.

As easy as it is for me to tell these stories as a joke, the fact is that every time these come-ons happened to me, my heart would start racing with a kind of wild primal fear. Yes, I am conflict averse and not at all good at politely shutting down an awkward situation. But there was much more to it than that. Women making advances just petrified me.

The few romantic relationships I have had with women have always started off safely. I met my wife Margie in high school and we only got together after she'd broken up with her boyfriend. My relationship with my partner Michelle started as an incredible friendship—true, it blossomed into romance while my marriage was falling apart, but there was nothing sudden or aggressive about it.

In some ways, Arlene was the exception. Up until I met her, I was completely terrified of talking to a strange woman! The first few times I told this to her, she laughed. But then one day, she asked me what I really meant by it. What that fear was all about.

Over the decade since then, I have been trying to piece together an answer. I hate to be all dramatic about this, but I'm pretty sure it started *in my childhood*.

Specifically, in third or fourth grade. Almost every day during recess on the playground, I would find myself surrounded by a group of girls, demanding to know which one of them I liked.

"Who's got the prettiest hair, Dick?"

"Who do you want to kiss?"

"Which one of us is your girlfriend?"

It may have seemed like innocent fun to the onlooking teachers who did nothing to stop it, but from my vantage point, trapped in the middle of that circle, it was utterly menacing. They wouldn't let me out until I answered their taunts, and no matter which name I spat out, that only seemed to make it worse during the next recess.

My next experience with this kind of powerless fear was even more unsettling. One day in fifth grade, my teacher asked me to stay after school. No explanation. When all the other kids had gone, it was just me and her, and she announced that she'd like my help grading her sixth graders' grammar quizzes. Well, I wasn't any good at fifth-grade grammar, much less sixth, so that made no sense at all.

She pulled a chair up next to her desk and patted it for me to come sit down beside her. I looked at that chair and I looked at her, and I knew something was wrong. This was not normal, and I was terrified.

Still, she was the teacher, so I took my seat beside her. She made a big show of pulling out the quizzes and showing me how to grade them, as if this was all standard procedure. When I struggled to do my "job," she moved in closer to help.

Finally, I kicked into escape mode and stood up from the chair. I sputtered some random lie—"I have to get home and watch my brother!" or "I forgot I have a dentist appointment!"—and shot out of that room as fast as I could. Never telling anyone about it for my whole life until I told Arlene.

At seventeen, I went to a college sorority dance and the singer for the band started making moves on me, hard. "Let's hit the road," she said to me. "Let's run away together!" Never mind that she was twice my age and I was there with a date!

I wiggled my way out of that one pretty easily, but my heart was pounding out of my chest, just like I was back in the playground or that classroom.

None of these incidents amount to anything like severe childhood sexual trauma; I'm not trying to claim that. Nor, in telling these stories, do I mean to downplay how truly destructive young trauma can be on the rest of one's life. But these were aggressions that scared the heck out of me, and that fear did stay inside me and build up.

Now that I see the pattern and say it out loud—I feel scared and cornered with women I don't know—it's a small but important relief. I can take my fear out of the category of "What the hell is that all about?" and put it in the category of "Okay, now I know why I'm a little weird." And when situations arise that trigger that fear again, I can breathe through it, see it as part of a pattern, and handle myself in it with more care.

Most of my fans, male and female, are incredibly respectful and gentle. But there are times when their emotions get the better of some of them, and they grab my hand too tightly or move in too close. Times when there's an intensity in their feelings for me that scares me. If Arlene or Jimmy aren't nearby to kindly steer them away, I do my best on my own. I ease back, release my hand with a smile, and redirect my attention.

All the while, breathing deliberately. I know my fear now, so I can control it.

HELP SOMEONE FIND THEIR VOICE: DO'S AND DON'TS

My own life has been full of great teachers and mentors, who helped me find "my voice" in performance. Starting with dear Mrs. Miller, who directed me in plays at Danville High School and then forty years later, came to see me in the revival of *The Music Man* and gave me notes after the show! Gower, Chita, and the whole cast of *Bye Bye Birdie* poured all their wisdom and talent into giving me a crash course in Broadway musicals, and of course Carl was my "head teacher" in television.

Much later in life, I found myself in the teacher-mentor role myself, with my wife Arlene, as she learned to sing. It was the most profound and moving experience of my entire later life. Helping her grow recalled my own old memories and feelings of growing.

It also helped me appreciate just how patient and generous my teachers had been. I tried to channel and model them, and I think I succeeded. But I also made some mistakes, which I have learned from.

It's important for me to tell this story from both my perspective and Arlene's, which is why you'll hear her words too. It has taught me not just what it means to be a mentor, but also what it means to find yourself.

After Arlene and I got married, our magical adventure really began. I don't mean travel. Ours was an adventure of discovering each other, growing into each other, and forging our own little culture of two.

Starting out, music was the place where we had the least in common. Arlene liked a lot of new stuff, and I had my old stuff. Now, I'm excited to explore a lot of uncharted territory in my life, but I can't say that her music was really piquing my curiosity. Except for Adele, who really takes me places.

Meanwhile, Arlene was much more open to broadening her horizons. And she had a thing called Spotify, which allowed her to hear, in their produced form, all the old tunes I was always humming around the house. Fats Waller, Jack Teagarden, Cy Coleman. New Orleans jazz.

Early on, I don't think I fully appreciated just how big of an undertaking this was for Arlene. She wouldn't have done it if she didn't really love what she was hearing, but she was literally digesting whole decades of all different genres of music. Including classical, which I adore, and all the songs from my movies and musicals! When I asked what was driving her, she said the most incredible thing: "I want to know what your life sounded like."

Quite naturally, she started singing along to these tunes around the house and in the car with me. She had always sung along to her own music before meeting me, but never in public (except for karaoke). But this felt a little more purposeful. I shared what I knew about the history of the songs, and we talked through all their layers of emotional meaning.

The more we explored the process of interpreting a song, *inhabiting* it, the more excited she got. Her voice found depth and nuance, and she was challenging herself to find true connection to each note and word. What had started as an effort just to understand her new husband's old world of music was fast becoming a passion for that music, a desire to know it by singing it.

For the first time in her life, Arlene was feeling and owning her voice. To me, it felt like singing was her way of discovering herself.

One night at home, she surprised me with a romantic cabaret: Nina Simone's "Feeling Good," Peggy Lee's "Fever." Imagine what this was like for me: the woman of my dreams is singing me love songs like they were written just for me!

What came next was my fault. I think we'd both agree that I got too excited about what was happening for Arlene and wanted to share it with the world.

The first occasion was a fundraiser at City Hall.

> ARLENE: We were going to do two songs. I wasn't a trained performer. I'd been trained by him and that was it. We had a pianist, which I was happy about, but they were kind of clunky. I didn't have the experience to notice at the time, but Dick sure did. We finished the first song, "An Old-Fashioned Wedding," which I had thought was fine, and Dick just kind of whisked us offstage. "Thank you, thank you," and that was it. We didn't do another song. I couldn't figure out what had gone wrong, and I didn't ask.

Honestly, to this day, I can't remember why I did that either. But the next one, Arlene reminds me, I was very specific.

It was the ninetieth birthday of Rose Marie, my beloved colleague from *The Dick Van Dyke Show*. Long before her adult acting career, Rose Marie was Baby Rose Marie, a child star who'd sung and performed on the radio and in film since she was three years old.

ARLENE: I decided to learn all these Baby Rose Marie songs from back when she was a kid. Eventually I picked "Take a Picture of the Moon" and practiced it a lot. This was a really big thing for me, to go out and talk and introduce the song and then sing it. Well apparently, I was off-key.

DICK: You were flat.

ARLENE: I don't know if I noticed Dick's face at the time, but then he comes out and we do "Carolina in the Morning" from *The Dick Van Dyke Show*, the first song I'd learned with him. That went fine. Then we did "Supercalifragilisticexpialidocious," which I didn't really know, so I was just kind of going along.

Well, afterward, he said to me directly: You were off-key. You were flat. And then—I mean, it was one of the harshest criticisms he ever gave me.

DICK: What did I say?

ARLENE: I barely remember myself. But I remember you said you should be embarrassed. That it was embarrassing.

DICK: Was I that harsh? I didn't yell, did I?

ARLENE: No. I've heard you yell, this was not yelling. But it did hurt my feelings.

DICK: I did?

ARLENE: You weren't letting up.

I'll be the first to admit that I am a tough critic. Whenever Arlene and I find ourselves captive to a subpar performance, I grouse to her under my breath: "Get off the stage." The stage is sacred to me, and you need to be good to get up there.

Also, as a teacher assessing their students' progress, it's not right to hold back the truth. If someone doesn't know they need to get better, how are they going to get better?

Arlene really gets that too. She says that if I had sugar-coated the truth with her about singing badly, then she'd never know if I was telling the truth about her singing well. She wanted to learn.

Still, this is the love of my life we're talking about, not a student. I could have said it another way. I didn't have to say "embarrassment."

It took some time for the sting to wear off, Arlene tells me, and then my critique had a motivating effect on her. It made her more determined when we practiced together.

Sure enough, it wasn't long before she stopped singing flat. And she could really hear the difference herself too. When that happened, her voice just opened up.

The Vantastix had a gig coming up at Disney's D23 fan convention, and I asked Arlene if she wanted to do a number with us onstage. Zero hesitation, she was all in.

It was a 1,500-person crowd, and with Arlene leading the way, we worked magic with the old Southern lullaby, "Didn't

Leave Nobody but the Baby." Her voice brought such warmth to our sound, and I loved having her up onstage with us. For me, it was just as easy and cozy as singing together at home. Understandably, Arlene was a bit more nervous than I was, but she really delivered.

That was it, we all agreed: Arlene brought something we needed, and she was with us to stay. Even when Arlene wasn't singing, she was listening. And let me tell you: There's no more perfect training for a vocalist than listening to, and singing along with, live a cappella and barbershop.

During that eternity of COVID lockdown, a lot of people in the world went full-on crazy. But not me and Arlene. That's when we truly started finding our voice as a duet. I mean, practically all we did during that time was find new songs to learn and explore together.

I'll never forget our experience with Ella Fitzgerald's "Blue Skies." On our first listen together, when Ella launches into her extended scat, I marveled aloud over how she could make such an impossible feat sound so effortless. I saw Arlene's eyes light up, now absorbing the song from the technical perspective of a singer. Then, unbeknownst to me, she went off and learned the whole thing, every single note, syllable, and growl! When she finally let me in on the results of all her hard work, I was just blown away. My wife could scat!

When Arlene's stepfather died, she decided she wanted to sing at the funeral instead of talking. A song was the best way she knew to share her love for her grieving mother and extended family.

Not just any song, either: she wanted to do "Amazing Grace." She sang it for me a few times at home, and it dawned on me she didn't have an accompanist lined up.

"So you're doing this *a cappella*?" I asked tentatively.

"Yup."

This was, I realized, a wise move. We both knew that a pianist, especially one you don't know, can really trip you up.

Before the funeral, the priest suggested that I do something, too, and he gave me a poem to read after Arlene's song: Tennyson's "Crossing the Bar," a funeral standard. I prepped it like a pro, but turns out, that didn't really matter.

When Arlene started to sing, you could feel the electricity just crackling through the crowd. Her voice, her whole being was radiant. She did incredible things with the tune, gathering and building the emotion as she went. I don't think anybody in the family had really known what a singer she'd become, so along with the feeling of the song, there was just this profound awe—at Arlene's sheer presence. By the end, the whole place was in tears. They even applauded—at a funeral!

She was an impossible act to follow, but I tried.

Afterward, there was a huge line of people pushing in to thank and hug Arlene and gush over her performance. A few folks noticed me at her side and nodded politely.

"Thanks for the poem."

REIMAGINE YOUR LEGACY

I've been back to my hometown of Danville, Illinois, on occasion in my later life. In 2004, I returned to accept a community honor and watch a student production of *Bye Bye Birdie* at my old high school. I sang and danced with the cast, which was a delight. And old classmates and friends showed up too—people I hadn't seen in years.

Most significantly, I got my high school diploma! Rather belatedly, I admit. At seventeen, I had left high school early to go into the military, then went into show business right after that, and basically never looked back. By age seventy-nine, I didn't need the cap-and-gown treatment, but Danville threw me a nice party.

Around 2015, I got some awful news from someone back home: the house I grew up in had been condemned and was about to be demolished. It hadn't been occupied since 2011 (seven years after my last visit) and had fallen into total disrepair. I wasn't prepared for the heartache I felt, and Arlene was just as distraught.

Danville's mayor got wind of the situation, grew worried that the house in fact had already been torn down, and dug into old records to figure out exactly which house it was. He called me up and said there was no abstract of title in the Van

Dyke name for my house, and I told him right away that it had been in my grandmother's name.

Yes, we had the right house and no, it hadn't been demolished yet. Whew.

Right away, we set up a foundation to buy the place and restore it. A local Realtor organized a volunteer effort to clear out some of the debris and at least keep the damaged parts from getting worse. They did an incredible job.

In 2016, Arlene and I went back to see the house and announce our plans to, eventually, turn it into a museum and a center for local young performing artists. In the Danville of my youth, performing arts had altered the course of my life. It felt natural to try and open up those doors for Danville's current youth population.

Like a lot of Midwestern towns, Danville had long been in a state of economic decline. But the spirit of the community was very much alive, as was the residents' drive to give their young people a brighter future there.

Our arrival in town was a joy. At a big town celebration, I sang and danced and performed with the high schoolers again. They unveiled (a surprise gift from Arlene) a funny custom traffic sign with my silhouette, walking, that bore the title of my last book (and my favorite maxim): KEEP MOVING.

When we went over to my old neighborhood, it was tough to see my childhood home so forlorn, but I could also imagine what it would look like fixed up, what it could become. As we stood in front, people streamed out of their houses, up and down the block, to come over and say hello.

"Nice to meet you!" I chirped, shaking hands awkwardly and pointing at the house. "I grew up here!"

"Hi there" or "Nice to meet you," some responded politely. "We heard about that."

Some people seemed weirded out about being in the presence of a celebrity, and others just seemed wary in general, and the overeager "showman" persona I fell into out of my own discomfort wasn't helping. The whole thing was shaping up to feel stiff and unnatural, all of us standing apart, none of us sure what to do or say.

Then, the crowd shifted and parted as someone—apparently someone important—moved through it from behind. Finally, a little old lady emerged with an air of intense emotion. She walked right up to me, reached out, wrapped her arms around me, and pulled me in for a long, deep hug.

With that, I felt my anxious formality just melt away. And you could feel the whole crowd around us relaxing too. Suddenly, our smiles were big and warm, and our body language was open and loose. People laughed, and we all started talking—naturally. Like neighbors.

I wish I had better news for what's happened since 2016.

Restoration plans have stalled and it's really looking like the house, at the end of the day, will be unsalvageable. The place is now turning into even more of an eyesore and a source of local frustration, which breaks my heart. I feel terrible that my old home is causing neighbors to worry about their property values and their safety. There still are plenty of local folks who want us to go forward with the museum and performing arts plans, but others just want the house gone.

Honestly, I don't know what we're going to do next. At ninety-nine, travel is almost impossible for me, so I can't go and do anything hands-on. And Arlene's plate is more than full, taking care of me. So far, we don't have anybody local that's really equipped or committed to take the endeavor on.

Back in 2016, I had dreamed that the arts center would be kind of my legacy: the thing I gave back to the community that had nourished me, an important piece of my heart that would live on after I die.

Maybe, though, it's better to think about my legacy in a different way. Not as something tied to a physical place, but rather as a spirit that will survive, in the body of my work and accomplishments, and in people's hearts.

Honestly, I don't care how long the memory of me, Dick Van Dyke, lasts in the world after I'm gone. I care about the survival of what I've shared with the world: humor, compassion, a zest for living, a love of music. For as long as children are proudly belting out their new word "Supercalifragilistic-expialidocious" or singing and skipping along to "Chim Chim Cher-ee," the most important part of me will always be alive.

READ THE FINE PRINT

I was married in 1948 and started to have a family right away, so I got life insurance. Term life insurance, to be exact. At the time, I didn't quite absorb what that meant. So, I turned ninety-five and I got a notice informing me that my policy had expired! What?! It was horrible. And God knows how much I had paid into the thing. Of course, I hadn't read the fine print, but who does?

Man oh man oh man. They got us coming and going, don't they?

LEARN FROM ANIMALS: 3 SPECIES, 4 RULES

On darker days when I'm in a "yelling at the TV" mood, I have been known to issue all sorts of proclamations that I haven't really thought through. This is one of my standards: "Hands down, animals are better than people!"

Okay, fine, sure. But what good is that going to do us humans, who need all the help we can get at being better?

Here's a more helpful way of phrasing that: "We humans could sure learn a lot from animals!"

My revised thesis reflects the fact that we humans are capable of growing and changing, which I'd say is much more where I really stand on the matter. And that nonhumans, in their nonhuman ways, can model and guide us in our ongoing evolution.

In my life, I have known and loved more animals than I can count. Dogs, cats, cows, coyotes, racoons, a chimp. I'm also the world's biggest fan of animal videos and nature shows. Watching nonhumans doing their thing is one of my greatest pleasures. If they're generous enough to rope me in on their thing, all the better, but that's not required. It's the observation and contemplation and reflection part that I really thrive on, when I get to wonder about their brains and spirits, and, hopefully, connect some of that back to my own experience as a human.

Consider some of my favorite animals, and the things they've shown me, or reminded me, about being a better human.

1. SHAKE OFF THE PAST: DIXIE AND TARZAN

When I was eleven or twelve, the Danville police station put Dixie, its German shepherd police dog, up for adoption because she was pregnant. Maybe taking her was my parents' idea, or maybe it was mine; however it happened, Dixie was now a member of the Van Dyke household, and I was her primary caretaker.

She was gorgeous. And she also was a local celebrity, so walking her around town gave me a swell of pride. Plus, I could not wait to see her puppies.

One day though, I was crossing the street with her and a car bumped her in the rump and knocked her off her feet. Anguished, I huddled over her until she could get to her feet. The vet said she wasn't badly hurt, but the accident might affect her pregnancy.

At that prognosis, my stomach dropped. I felt so guilty and so worried.

Not long after that, back at home, Dixie slunk down under the back porch and didn't come out. Which, I gathered from my parents, meant she was ready to give birth.

Of course, I needed to be right by her side. I sat there on that porch, waiting, ducking down to peer into the dark, waiting and waiting. Somebody asked me to go to a football game and I said, "No, I'm staying with Dixie."

Eventually, the painful silence from under the porch gave way to new movement, and I scuttered under there as close as I could get to Dixie. Who was licking at something that was moving down at her belly.

A single puppy. Half German shepherd, half I don't know what. A mystery mongrel.

Once the puppy had its footing, it came crawling out from under the porch so I could really meet it. But as soon as daylight hit its face, that mongrel was growling, snarling and biting at my fingers. He'd been born mad and hated life from the get-go.

My heart sank. The survivor had not emerged unscathed.

Still, I kept up hope. I named him Tarzan, praying there was something else in him besides savage.

Sure enough, over the weeks and months to come, Tarzan stopped lunging and raging at me like I was to blame for all his misery, and he came to appreciate that maybe I was half decent. He never was warm and cuddly, nor was he particularly active, but he did settle into life. Knowing how close he had come to not being alive at all, I considered that a victory.

Dixie did alright herself, and together, we'd sit and watch Tarzan in the backyard like a regular couple of parents. Every now and then, a squirrel or a stranger, or even me on his grumpier days, would send Tarzan back into the hateful mode of his youth, snapping with murder in his eyes.

Oh no, I'd think. Bad Tarzan back. And it's all my fault.

Then, once the drama had passed, he'd do this thing that all dogs do, but to me at the time, was a new revelation. That full-body shake-it-off thing, like a factory reset. The upsetting event that had just happened was now gone, and a fresh new little chapter of life was getting started.

2. GIVE DIRECTIONS TO A LOST STRANGER: PORPOISES OF THE ATLANTIC OCEAN

In the 1940s, Phil and I were doing our Merry Mutes act at a club in Virginia Beach. We performed at night, so our days were free. Ambling down the boardwalk by myself one afternoon, I spotted a surf shop, advertising board rentals and lessons.

Back in LA, I had tried surfing and liked it a lot—it was the perfect way to forget about something (the struggle of my life) by focusing on something else (the waves). Doing comedy club to club was grueling, and for a couple hours, I was happy to forget it. One of those big ten-foot boards would do just the trick.

The waves of the Atlantic were meager compared to the Pacific, and I quickly lost the energy and enthusiasm to catch them. Instead, I paddled out beyond the breakers and gave in to my deep-bone exhaustion, lying flat on my board and falling asleep in the sun.

Here's how long I slept, which is also how tired I was: when I woke up, there was no land in sight. Not kidding. All I saw was gentle ocean, in every direction, and the sun, a lot farther down and closer to the horizon.

Well, at least I knew which way was west-ish. I started paddling, hoping to soon feel a clear current pulling me toward shore.

No sir, I was in deep water. Which meant a lot more paddling to come. I had energy from the long nap and the boyish excitement of being "at sea," but there was also a stab of worry. Exactly how long would I have to keep paddling? What happens when the sun goes down?

Suddenly, I felt a bump from underneath my board. Flotsam? Then another. Flotsam-jetsam?

Then the bumps became regular. This was not debris. This was something alive, underneath me.

A fin broke water right beside me, then another behind it, and of course, my mind screamed: *Shaaaaark!* and I prepared to be chomped.

Then, the owners of these fins made themselves visible and I could see they were a pod of porpoises. Harmless, playful porpoises, just having a bit of fun with a splashing stranger.

Or maybe something else? They were bumping me with purpose, with direction! And that direction was westward, toward the sun, toward the shore!

Which, maybe five minutes into this bumping and pushing, I could finally glimpse for myself. Breathing a sigh of relief, I resumed my paddling, all the while gladly accepting the porpoises' continued bumps of guidance and momentum.

Eventually, because they no doubt had something better to do with their time, they darted off and left me to reach shore on my own. Gliding onto the sand, I leaped to my feet practically bouncing with glee. When I turned back to the ocean, there were no fins in sight to thank, but I did so anyway.

My rational mind told me that the porpoises had any number of biologically appropriate reasons for their behavior. Maybe they were following fish and I just happened to be in their path of feeding. Maybe they were, in fact, just bumping for fun, which also tangentially was guiding me to shore.

But I saw the whole thing more magically. The pod detected a land creature in the sea, which meant it wasn't where it belonged, and they were returning it toward its rightful home. Like if you saw a toddler toddling too close to a campfire: you step in and steer it in the other direction.

How effortless this little intervention is for whoever's doing it! And how crucially important for whoever's receiving it! You can make a person's day, or save a person's life, just with a moment of help. All it takes is noticing that they need it.

3. MAKE IT BACK HOME: TORNADO CAT AND BOBO

In 1954, I took a new job with a Louisiana TV station and uprooted the growing Van Dyke family—Margie (pregnant with Stacy), Chris, Barry, and two Siamese cats—from Atlanta to New Orleans. It was hard for us to move again, just a few years into our life in Atlanta, which we'd hoped would be more or less permanent.

We had one another, which helped make wherever we went together feel like home. And we also had those two cats, who worked as a kind of a "transitional object" for the boys, like a security blanket or a stuffed animal. I have squeezed at my brain until I have a headache to remember those cats' names, but I just can't. True to their breed, they chatted and caterwauled nonstop, craved human affection and companionship, and cast a spell over the whole family with their wild blue eyes. Even me, who always liked dogs much better.

Our new house was on a wide street with a big grassy mall in the middle, and when the cats weren't inside entertaining us, they were out there frolicking and hunting. One weekend afternoon, the sky turned dark-greenish and the wind suddenly picked up. Our first big New Orleans storm was coming in fast, so the whole family gathered inside by the front window to watch. The two cats were still out in the grass and about to get soaked.

Well, they got more than soaked. It only took a second for Margie and I to realize that this wasn't just a thunderstorm: the wind was roaring, ripping branches off trees and rattling the whole house. Just as the hunch entered our minds, it was confirmed right out our window. Garbage cans, trees and stop signs were in the air, along with every other thing unlucky to be caught in the tornado's path. The boys screamed the cats' names, then a great whoosh splattered our window with so much water that whatever was happening outside was now, mercifully, invisible.

Not thirty seconds later, it was all over. Margie and I hurried outside to see a clean path of devastation, right down the middle of the street, just four or five blocks long. No house on either side was damaged, but that stretch of middle ground, where the tornado had touched down, was just torn to pieces.

The cats were nowhere in sight. Given what Margie and I had actually seen, it was impossible for us not to imagine what we hadn't seen: the two Siamese, swirling up into the funnel. It was horrifying.

Much harder was fielding the barrage of questions from our anguished boys over the next many days. "We don't know what happened to them." "They may have found a place to hide." "We'll call everyone we know." "We'll go looking." "They may come home on their own." "We'll just have to wait."

Every day, the boys put food out on the front porch, hoping to entice the cats home. We got a lot of stray free-loaders, but no Siamese. The house felt painfully quiet without those weird feline moans. Losing the cats kind of unmoored us all, at a time when mooring was just what we needed. Maybe we should get a new pair of Siamese, Margie and I wondered aloud.

Then, weeks later, miracle of miracles: a familiar meow, long and desperate. Hovering at a window was one of the cats, wanting inside!

As soon as we opened the door, it shot past our legs and under the cover of furniture. No amount of coaxing would bring it out for a welcome-home cuddle. When it was finally too hungry to hide, it came out for food, and we noticed that half of one ear had been torn off.

A trip to the vet is traumatizing for any cat, but for one who's also fresh out of a tornado, it must be so much worse. The physical wound healed easily, but the cat remained a total nervous wreck. Its meows felt all jumbled; they didn't have their old meanings. It wouldn't come near us and stopped coming inside at all. It was always starting and jerking at phantom threats. In short, the cat seemed to have gone nuts.

We felt abandoned by this new personality, and it seemed likely that the other cat was gone for good—a double blow. Margie gave birth to Stacy and a new baby sister worked wonders keeping the boys' minds off our feline tragedy.

Alone sometimes, I'd watch our survivor outside, flailing for the threads of its old self. Following a familiar path in the grassy plaza, then swerving off. Batting at objects that wouldn't move. It was a painful sight.

But when I considered the bigger picture, I realized that we had more of a miracle story on our hands. Imagine what that cat must have been through! How high it must have been sucked, how far it must have been tossed. And after all that, still managing to find its way home, which had only been its home for a matter of months!

That crazy cat was not to be pitied. It was to be admired!

Just last December, I was reminded of our old Siamese Odysseus during another natural disaster: the Franklin Fire, which swept down toward our Malibu home in the dead of night at a terrifying speed, triggering a panicked community wide evacuation.

We had been through the Woolsey Fire in 2018 (and I'd been through fire evacuations before that), so we thought we were all prepared, ready to flee in a moment's notice. Arlene had no trouble collecting our dog and three cats, but locating the cat *carriers* was a frantic scramble. Note to reader: Keep animal carriers accessible and close to the door.

Meanwhile, I waged and lost an exhausting battle with the water hose, struggling to give our backyard a last-minute dousing before we escaped. I was so wiped out that I kind of had to crawl on my way out to the car, and then some neighbors came and carried me.

Arlene managed to wrangle all the carriers and animals . . . Except, right at the last minute, Bobo, our dear tabby, shot off—nowhere to be found. Embers were flying, the smoke was thickening: we had no choice but to speed away and leave Bobo behind.

At two in the morning, we arrived at the Georgian Hotel in Santa Monica to get a room. The man who stumbled into that posh lobby in no way resembled anyone's vision, past or present, of Dick Van Dyke. I was dripping wet, no shirt and a sheepskin jacket, barefoot, Arlene slogging in with me, her arms full of cat carriers. We looked insane.

For the next two days, we hovered over the TV set in the room. I couldn't sleep at all, which meant I was *feeling* insane now too. Hour after hour, we agonized over the fate of our beloved home, which was a total unknown, and also Bobo. Of course, this reminded me of losing and worrying over those tornado cats in New Orleans, but I kept it to myself. Arlene knows that story and hates it, and it would be the opposite of helpful.

When Arlene posted a note on social media that we were safe, but Bobo was missing, suddenly "Bobo the Missing Cat" became a headline story. Pictures of his adorable sad orange face were everywhere! Meanwhile, news trucks were broadcasting from our neighborhood, and we could see our neighbor's house burning to the ground. Frustratingly, we couldn't see any angles that showed our house.

Both of us feared the worst. I had lived in that house since the 1980s. It contained all my earthly possessions, my entire life. It was too horrific to even imagine all of it being lost.

We made it back home as soon as we possibly could. The place was safe, but just barely. The fire had come right up to the edge of our property, burned our Halloween stage and scorched the back of one of our outbuildings. But thanks to the heroic efforts of our neighbors Alec, Kent, and Abel, who had stayed through the fire, watering the perimeters of everyone's properties to keep the fire at bay, nothing else was damaged. I wept with exhausted relief; I loved and cherished our little house and everything in it. I depended on being there to feel safe, to feel myself.

And look, who's that waiting out in the backyard? Hero cat miracle number two: it's Bobo! Who, we realized, had probably never even left our property. He was physically fine but loudly upset at being left alone—I imagine he'd had quite the fright seeing and feeling the fire so close. He didn't give a damn about our physical and emotional upheaval, nor did he care that his survival was a feel-good story in the news.

Meanwhile, for days after our return, all I did was weave around the house, twitching at shadows and caterwauling nonsensically for Arlene. Tornado Cat, I really feel you.

4. FIND A PURPOSE FOR EVERYONE: ROCKY AND THE KITTENS

After my partner Michelle died, Rocky, our wire hair fox terrier, fell into deep grief right alongside me. When Arlene came into my life, she was a cat person, so it took her a while to warm up and surrender to Rocky's unquenchable need for love and affection.

Late in life, Rocky was remarkably resilient. His hind legs went, and we got him one of those little two-wheel things so he could still move around. He hated it, but he made it work. At the time, we had just gotten these four orange rescue kittens, and Rocky took them in like he was their mother. He would watch over them as they ate, groom them, and herd them together if they wandered astray.

Those kittens brought Rocky alive again. When he was old and feeble and feeling useless, they gave him purpose.

Once, we put Rocky up on the bed with the kittens, not sure what would happen. Well, it turns out mothering is a two-way street. They all just huddled around him like a team of nurses, nuzzling and licking and taking care of him. Then he'd lick them back, and they'd lick him some more.

What a beautiful thing, the simple act of caring for another being. Giving and getting love, a fully mutual pleasure.

GET A GOOD DJ

October 2024. The Van Dyke household was in a state of complete mayhem. My grandkids were running around, my kids were running around after my grandkids, and there were swarms of people I didn't know too. A lighting crew, a sound crew, a film crew, and a Malibu neighbor you may have heard of: Chris Martin, the lead singer and cofounder of Coldplay.

They were here to shoot a video for the band's song "All My Love," with Spike Jonze directing, and me in front of the camera. The video was envisioned as kind of a love letter to me and my life, in honor of my ninety-ninth birthday. I would sit at the piano in the backyard with Chris while he played and sang to me, and that would be intercut with moments of me reminiscing, celebrating with my family, and dancing barefoot, which is my favorite thing to do.

It was a beautifully simple concept, as Chris had described it, a pure expression of his affection for me. He was a huge *Mary Poppins* fan, and we had long been friendly, but there was something so tender and intimate about his vision for the project, it really melted my heart. I was honored and inspired.

And I wanted to give it, and him, my best.

The biggest hurdle, I am sorry and embarrassed to admit, was the music. Arlene had played the song for me several times, so I could get in the mood. It's an aching ballad, and Arlene loves it.

I trust her implicitly, but at my core, I'm just not a ballad kind of person. And I really couldn't "hear" the song—as in feel a way into the flow of the music.

Without that, how could I dance to it?

Arlene gently relayed this back to the production team and suggested a workaround, using music that I knew and loved instead for the dancing scenes.

Problem solved. Except once we started shooting, there I was in the backyard, bare feet at the ready, and they put on "All My Love." The cameras were rolling and they're looking at me, waiting for me to break out some moves, and absolutely nothing was coming to me.

I was trying my very best to feel it, but I couldn't. The last thing I wanted to do was let Chris down, but my body would not move.

Fortunately, my little struggle only lasted a few moments before Arlene stepped in and took charge.

"I'm sorry, Chris. I love the song," she said. "But he can't hear it. It's too slow for him."

With that, she huddled with the sound guy, pulled up a whole roster of songs she knew would get me moving . . . and found the perfect one.

Because this is always what Arlene does.

She's seen how stiff I am during photo shoots; how hard it is for me to just pose and look great on command with nothing in the way of inspiration. She says I'm like one of those roadside air puppet guys on a windless day. So, she's taken to putting on some New Orleans music, and voilà, I'm bouncing and shimmying and waving to all the passersby.

The song she picked for me on this day, however, was even more perfect—because it came with a personal backstory.

Back in 1959 or 1960, I auditioned for *Bye Bye Birdie*. With scant musical theater experience and no formal dance training at all, I felt totally unprepared. But the director Gower Champion wanted to see me dance, so I had to at least try. And the only way I could even try was with a song I loved. "Once in Love with Amy" is a soft, sweet number that just makes you want to sway and soft-shoe as you sing. So that's just what I did.

And Gower gave me the part on the spot, despite me then admitting point-blank that I couldn't dance! He'd teach me, he said. That part won me a Tony and it changed my life. And "Once in Love with Amy" has remained one of my favorites ever since.

So, when I heard those melancholy opening chords, all that memory and meaning came flooding back to me. I got right into it and my feet started moving, then my arms and whole body, and I couldn't stop.

There was a spotlight on me, and Arlene says it was like watching a movie. She says she's never seen my body move like that before.

WRITE IT DOWN

If you're like me, you have great ideas that pop up at the most inopportune moments and then disappear just as quickly. Like you're at the eye doctor staring at an anatomical illustration of the inside of an eyeball and you get a vision for a new Halloween mask. By the time the eye appointment is over, the mask idea is long gone.

What's left, instead, is the memory of having inspiration, which you then spend far too much time trying to conjure back up. Occasionally, a forgotten idea will pop in later and you vow this time that you'll remember it for sure, and then, whoosh, it's gone again.

This goes on for your whole life and at certain points, you stop and reflect sadly back on all the amazing stuff you've just let fizzle out of your brain and into the ether. Not the specifics, of course, because you don't remember what those are, but the totality of them in absence.

This kind of thing would never happen if you were Marge Mullen.

Marge was the script supervisor for the full run of *The Dick Van Dyke Show* (and *The Mary Tyler Moore Show* and so many shows after that too!). The job of script supervisor is more like a dozen jobs rolled into one, and Marge did them all with rigor and a brilliant ear for humor.

She was most treasured for her unfailing ability to write everything down. And I do mean everything. When Carl, the writers, and cast were brainstorming our shows together, we'd throw out all kinds of ideas, for stories, characters, plot twists, lines and bits of comedy.

Marge was always there, scribbling away whatever we blurted out, and then later, typing it all up. If we happened to be popping out ideas over lunch, Marge would be one table over, writing on a napkin.

I remember Marge most for the SOS.

While some of our ideas were stinkers, plenty had real potential. But we just couldn't work them into that particular show.

So, Marge created the SOS—"Some Other Show"—a big book in which she recorded all our "almost" ideas in rich detail. It was an amazing resource. At times when we were coming up dry, we'd flip through the SOS for stuff to pluck out.

I don't know what ever happened to the SOS, but I bet it has a full season of good material, just waiting to come to life.

SOS, Marge! Where's the SOS?!

Now, an SOS might not be able to bring *The Dick Van Dyke Show* back to life, but it's not too late for the rest of humanity. If each one of us kept an SOS, a record of all the incredible, transformative things that are possible for us to do, we'd be one step closer to actually doing them.

For instance, if I were to start my own SOS, I'd fill it up with a lot more than Halloween ideas. I'd put all the little nuggets of wisdom I wish I'd told my grandkids and all my ideas for presents for Arlene. I'd punch up my punch lines, record dreams that bewildered me but also felt important, list out the few working actors who could credibly play a good clown instead of just another evil one. I'd lay out my plan for making music education a national priority in public schools. I'd write down all my strategies for getting politicians to care, all of the ways we can help our neighbors being swallowed alive by hatred. I would write a catchy little song that tells a funny story, but also makes the case for kindness.

BOND THROUGH CRISIS

It was the middle of the night, and I was up yet again, throwing off all the blankets and pulling myself out of bed into the cold. Barefoot, I stumbled out into the dark house, clicking on my little flashlight to guide my path. Down the hall into the living room.

From there, it was a straight shot to the sliding glass doors, but I managed to crash into a few things en route nonetheless. I yanked the door open, and the gusts hit me. I hurried out onto the brick patio, as fast as a ninety-nine-year-old can hurry.

At the edge of the patio, I squinted up to the crest of the ridge. My eyes aren't great, but they're good enough to spot a fire. So far, there was no pale orange brightness and nothing in the way of an up-close orange-red line either.

Catching my breath, I stood there and squinted into the dark, trying to detect any emerging glow.

"Dick!"

Arlene was behind me. I guess she heard the crash.

"The fire isn't over there! It's coming from the Palisades!"

I absorbed this. I was looking in the wrong direction, the direction the last fire had come from, less than a month earlier.

"You're gonna freeze!" Arlene said.

She was right. I had all my clothes on because I'd been sleeping in them, but the air was bone-chilling.

She took me back inside, guided me back to bed, put all the blankets on top of me again, and told me to go to sleep. But we both knew I'd be up again in another hour.

A day earlier, on January 7, 2025, an unstoppable fire had engulfed practically the entire community of the Pacific Palisades. Now it was surging westward into southern Malibu. Meanwhile, another fire had broken out on the east side of Los Angeles and would destroy dozens of entire blocks in Altadena.

And yet, here we were at home. When we got the evacuation orders and the power went out, I had refused to go. This was the fifth major California fire I'd been through (if I'm counting correctly), including the Franklin Fire, which we had fled just weeks earlier. I just couldn't do it again. As I saw it, the trauma of leaving was as likely to kill me as a fire.

Arlene got it right away. I needed to be home. So, we decided to hunker down and wait and watch it out. Thankfully, Jimmy insisted on staying with us. When the Franklin Fire hit, they'd been on their way home to Burbank, and it was impossible to turn back. Now, we were all three together for however long this crisis was going to last.

Apparently, on that first night of me running outside every other hour, I had been leaving the sliding glass door open, which meant our animals might get out. So, Arlene asked Jimmy to sleep on the couch in the living room and keep watch in case I did it again. And to ease my fears about an encroaching fire, she drove me out to the Pacific Coast Highway. Looking down the coast, the sky was full of orange and smoke, but far in the distance. Having that visual reassurance was the only way I could get any sleep at all.

Still, I'd often pop awake, freezing cold because my pile of blankets had fallen to the floor. At my age, pulling oneself out of bed to scoop up a pile of blankets is no small feat, and being winded like that, over and over, left me weak and exhausted.

In addition to cutting off our power, the city cut off our gas, which meant our gas-powered generator was useless. Fortunately, our good neighbor Abel (true to his name in every sense and spelling) had power from his own propane tank. So, we ran a cord from his house to ours, which allowed us limited and intermittent electricity, too.

Portable heaters kept us warm. Huddling over them with Arlene and Jimmy, I couldn't help but recall winter mornings in my childhood: my mother, brother, and I standing on our personal floor vents waiting for the heat to come up from the coal furnace.

Two days in, Arlene and Jimmy ventured out to find gas for Arlene's car, which was almost empty. They came back home in a state of shock. They'd driven down the Pacific Coast Highway, right past the fires still raging, taking one oceanside house after another. It was like a monster, Arlene said.

We had a cupboard full of food and ended up going through almost all of it. Arlene would take her ingredients outside to her little pull-along Happier Camper and do all the cooking in there on a two-burner hot plate. She would come back bearing the most incredible meals, which always took me and Jimmy by surprise. How she was able to get that creative, I have no idea. We tried to eat our dinners before sunset, but sometimes we ate later in the dark, the table aglow from battery-powered discs and globes.

In lieu of hot water showers, we took hot towel baths, courtesy of Arlene's handy aesthetician's towel warmer. And luckily, we had some DVDs and a functioning DVD player, which meant I finally got to see *Elf*. What a delight! But wait a second—Bob Newhart and Ed Asner were in it, why hadn't they cast me?

As the days of blackout rolled on, being away from home got hard on Jimmy. Their partner Robin was at home in Burbank, living through the crisis alone. Robin is immunocompromised, and those winds were blowing smoke and ash all over Los Angeles, so she was pretty much trapped inside. She and Jimmy talked on the phone a lot, but still, it was agony for them.

Arlene was fielding calls constantly from friends and family checking in to make sure we were okay. Inevitably, people would ask why we hadn't evacuated, and Arlene would have to patiently explain our reasoning. She started doing live videos every day, to keep people posted on how we were doing.

The specifics of those eleven days are a blur to me now. But what sticks with me is the feeling we shared of living through that crisis, our little family of three hunkered down together. As ragged and shocked as we all were, we looked out for one another, each in our own ways. On instinct, we knew how important it was to keep our spirits up, so we sang, told stories, and made each other laugh as much as we could.

All of Los Angeles was like that too. In the aftermath of the fires, there was a mass outpouring of pure generosity, people opening their homes to traumatized strangers who'd lost everything, volunteering, donating food, clothing and money. It was as if, all at once, we realized how much we need one another to survive.

I hope we don't forget that.

Arlene and I will never leave our Malibu home, and that means we'll always live with the increasing dangers of climate change. More fires bring more mudslides, and it will keep going like this forever.

When I tell the stories of all my lucky escapes from fire, friends always joke that when "the apocalypse" hits, they'll come to stay with me.

Well, the apocalypse has already hit. And it's a permanent part of our future.

Hold each other tight.

BE SOMEONE'S BAKER

As bigger things like travel, walking, and making plans become harder in my advanced age, I tend to savor the smaller, more immediate pleasures instead. Like taste.

Jimmy's partner Robin seems to know this instinctively, maybe because she and Jimmy grew up in multigenerational homes and were very connected to their grandmothers. Or maybe it's because she's seen me around a dessert.

Jimmy says I'm like a hummingbird, which I guess means I hover eagerly over any sweet stuff on the table, then dive in, beak-first. I've always been like this, but it's really gotten out of control these past few years.

See, Robin has a surprise talent up her sleeve. In addition to loving Jimmy and somehow knowing all my old music backward and forward, she's a baker! And I am the drooling guinea pig for all her new recipes. Each week, she'll bake up some new dessert or pastry at home, then send it with Jimmy over to our house, where I will enjoy and evaluate it (Arlene, too, if she's quick). Then Jimmy will report my verdict back to Robin, and if it's a success, she'll put it in rotation.

Almost everything so far has been a big hit: cherry turnovers, banana bread, blueberry buckle, fudge, and all kinds of cookies. When she started her gooseberry pie, Robin was iffy about the recipe, and I'm glad my honest feedback has ensured that the pie will not be coming back.

I realize my role as "taste tester" is not exactly essential to Robin's growth as a baker, but I'm more than happy to keep up our little ritual.

Now, you may be wondering how eating sweets on a regular basis might qualify as a "rule" for living to one hundred. This rule isn't about what I'm doing. It's about what Robin is doing! And it's aimed at all of you who might have an elderly person like me in their life whose world is rapidly shrinking and whose pleasures are increasingly humble.

You don't have to be a baker. You could be a person with a driver's license who enjoys automotive meandering. A musician who could use a captive audience, a bookworm who wants to read aloud, a puzzler who needs a partner, a chatty phone chatter. Trust me: whoever you are, you have the skills for this job.

Based on what I have learned through my informal "Practicing Elder Kindness Through Pastries" mentorship with Robin, I have three simple guidelines for those of you embarking on your own journeys as practitioners.

1. Go with Your Gut

- Share something you already love.
- Keep your kindness simple and deliver it simply.
- Don't overthink anything—the stakes are low!

2. Make It Interactive

- Ask questions.
- Invite feedback and adjust accordingly.

- Make it a "doing" thing, together, and let them lead, if they want to (I don't want to bake; I just want to eat).

3. Keep Coming Back

- Make it regular; something for them to look forward to.
- If you're getting "no," adjust and keep trying.
- Even if you don't always get a "thank you," trust that you are appreciated.

Now, if after all this, you're still wondering "Yes, but how does practicing elder kindness get *me* to one hundred?" well I don't know what to tell you.

Actually, I do.

If you play a part in helping someone enjoy their older age, then you are automatically awarded ten to twenty years to your own lifespan, depending on how much they like your cookies. Robin receives thirty.

GET FRANK: A MEDITATION ON OLD RIFTS

On a bookshelf in my living room, there's a series of beautifully leather-bound scrapbooks from my early career. Whenever I look at them, I think of Frank Adamo, the dear man who made them for me. At first, this gives me a warm feeling, but then, inevitably, comes a stab of long-festering pain.

I first met Frank back in the early 1960s at an ad agency where I did some commercials. He worked there and we became friendly. He was a tall, lanky guy with a face full of character that you just couldn't forget. Not long after, Frank lost that job and came to me for help, waiting outside my rehearsal for *Bye Bye Birdie* in the February snow. He asked if I needed a dresser, a job I didn't know existed, and then he immediately proceeded to make himself indispensable—not just maintaining my wardrobe, but managing my schedule, running lines, you name it.

He came with me to *The Dick Van Dyke Show* as my assistant and (because we were the same height and build) my stand-in. But with Frank's look, thick New Yawk accent and comic timing, he belonged in front of the camera. Over the course of our five-year run, he popped up in a ton of episodes, playing one hilarious cameo oddball after another. There's even a Facebook fan page devoted to ranking his roles, including:

- A telegram messenger who sings a prank insult message to Rob in perfect bored deadpan.
- An effete lisping poet.
- A very serious avant-garde actor who recites nonsense lines to his scene partner, a watermelon: "Up! Down! Stay! Go!"

As essential as Frank was to the efficient day-to-day operation of my work, he also became a close friend. He helped steer me through my worries and struggles on the job and kept me grounded when I got scrambled. He also became part of my family, always on hand with eccentric birthday presents for the kids, sharing a warm friendship with my wife Margie.

When I got hired for *Mary Poppins*, Frank came along too. "He's part of the package," I told the studio.

Our director was a heavily accented British guy who pronounced Frank's name as "Frink."

"Frink!" he'd shout when it was time for Frank to stand in. "Frink!"

We all thought that was hilarious, and after a while, that's what we called him, too. Even my kids, who were sometimes around on set.

In addition to Frank's work for me, he did a brief stand-in for Julie Andrews. In one fleeting shot in the movie, you can see him, as Mary Poppins herself, flying up in the air with her dark hat and coat and umbrella.

Frank came to Europe for *Chitty Chitty Bang Bang*, and to Arizona when Margie and the kids and I moved out there in the early '70s. On the weekends, when Frank wasn't working for me on a show or special I was taping in the studio, he ran a little antique store in town. And then later, back in LA, Mary Tyler Moore hired him for her show, and he was with her for fifteen years.

Eventually, Frank met the love of his life and moved down to Florida, where they devoted their retirement to one of Frank's abiding passions: set and artistic design for theater. He designed, built, and painted backdrops, did lighting and created props, becoming just as beloved and indispensable in that world as he had been with me and Mary.

When Margie got sick with pancreatic cancer in 2007 (long after we had divorced), Frank would call from Florida and check in on how she was doing. She died in 2008, and I was a wreck, along with all our children.

In my scattered grief, I tried to call everyone who had known Margie, but somehow I forgot to call Frank. When he found out, he was so hurt and angry, and I'm not sure if he ever forgave me.

In the years after that, I would sometimes wonder if I should try to call him and apologize again. Then I worried that that might just reopen the wound. We ended up never speaking again, and Frank died in 2018. Now I still feel horrible about the whole thing, but there's nothing I can do.

I missed my chance at reconciliation. I guess we both did. And I wish we hadn't.

The other day, Arlene went rooting around in a box of old stuff and retrieved a clipping of a Florida newspaper article about Frank from 2002 (before our falling out), which I guess he'd either sent me or Margie, I'm not sure.

"Set Designer Recalls Sitcom Years," it's titled, with a big picture of Frank, now bald and goateed, very seriously stapling scenery. In the article, he recalls working for me and Mary with great fondness, and talks about how fulfilling his life in theater has been since then.

"If you're going to retire," he says at the end, "retire to do something you really like." As Arlene read that part, I broke into a smile. Now that's some advice that I can really get behind.

In lieu of actually being able to reconcile, that clipping has given me some peace about Frank. Instead of reliving our rift ad nauseum, I can now think of him enjoying his life. And, in particular, I can happily imagine one very colorful detail mentioned in the story: a set element that Frank had been designing at the time, for a production of *Mame*. A gold lamé moon.

REMEMBER THE GOOD STUFF, LEAVE THE REST BEHIND

"For the past few days," I announced one morning, "I've been wondering why there's a hole in my memory where Faye Dunaway used to be. Didn't I do a whole play on TV with her?"

Arlene and Jimmy looked up from whatever they were doing in the kitchen.

"Well, that's probably for the best," Arlene said.

"Definitely," Jimmy chimed in.

Hmmm. Was it that bad? Naturally, I was tempted to ask them to fill me in on the forgotten details.

But then I thought better of it. Did I really want to remember whatever it was they didn't want to tell me? *I'm ninety-nine years old! Do I really care anymore?*

I sat down at the table, and when it became clear I was not going to dig for dirt, Arlene and Jimmy breathed a silent sigh of relief.

Still, my mind couldn't quite get over its curious picking. And suddenly, there was Faye's impossibly gorgeous face, gazing intensely into my eyes, on the verge of issuing a Momentous Proclamation. This: the only true memory I have of her at all.

"I do recall that she once told me I must always wear white because I look good in it," I said. "So, every time I put on white, I feel like Faye is giving me a little nod of approval."

I gestured to my white tunic proudly, and Jimmy and Arlene chuckled.

"She's right," Arlene said, delivering my breakfast.

REMINISCE WHILE YOU CAN

Back in the '90s and early 2000s, I'd be flipping through the channels and stop on an old episode of *The Dick Van Dyke Show* that, for the life of me, I couldn't remember. We did 158 episodes from 1961 to 1965, so I guess that's no surprise.

So, I'd call up my dear old friend Carl Reiner, who created and wrote the show. Surely, he would remember.

"Hi, Dick."

"Turn on the TV, Carl."

He'd flip to the right channel, and I'd let him watch for a second to get his bearings.

"Do you remember this one?" I'd ask.

Carl would watch a bit longer. Sometimes, he'd remember the episode. But if it was one I didn't remember, it was usually one he didn't remember either.

So, we'd sit there on the phone together, watching the show as if it were brand-new. Both of us cracking up at the best bits. Reliving, as spectators, the sheer joy of our collaboration, without saying a word.

I guess you'd call this our way of reminiscing.

Now, three decades later, Carl has been gone from this world for five years. I can't pick up the phone and call him, so I'm left to reminisce about our reminiscing.

I miss him so much. I'll take what I can get.

GET A GREAT SIDEKICK

I don't know what it is about my assistant Jimmy that brings out my mischievous side, but I sure am grateful for it. It started as soon as they first came to work for me and Arlene.

Wait, *they*? Yes, I asked that, too, when we first met. Jimmy is forty-one, queer and trans, and their pronouns are they/them, all of which took some getting used to. These kids sure do keep us our toes, don't they?

Now where was I?

Maybe three days into Jimmy's new job, I decided it was time to test the waters in their humor department, so to speak. So I invited Jimmy to try the pool slide. Swimming's not really their thing, but I insisted. They dutifully did the slide, hit the water with a big splash, and I ran over, looking around in the rippling water, all wide-eyed.

"Is everything okay, Dick?" Jimmy said from the pool.

"Just checking to see if there's any water left in there!" I ribbed.

Sometimes we're all out at restaurants where there's live music. And I have a thing about piano players that get in the way of singers. They play the singer's part for them, or they start doing all this fancy stuff that overpowers the vocals. Maybe it's because they know I'm there and they want to show off.

"Why is he playing so much?" I'll grouse.

"Stop!" Arlene will whisper, reminding me that we're not watching TV at home.

So, then I'll just look over at Jimmy and do my most exaggerated faces of total disgust to make them crack up. Again, Arlene has to shush the kids.

I really got Jimmy once with a version of a prank I pull on Arlene. One morning, they arrived at our house for work and spotted my glasses "fallen" on the floor by the front door. So, they picked them up, cleaned them off and took them into my bedroom to return them to me. There, in my bed, was a horrifically desiccated corpse staring right at them. Jimmy screeched!

And then realized what it was. I like to keep a creepy old man mannequin lying around the house, and I'm always dressing it up and layering gruesome masks on its face to keep the look fresh. It's good for scaring off any potential intruders and also situations like this. Before Jimmy arrived, I'd carried it into my bedroom and tucked it into my bed just perfectly.

"I thought something horrible had happened!" Jimmy said later. "Your face was melted!"

During the early days of COVID, Jimmy took me to the pharmacy to get some medications. This was before a vaccine, everybody was squirrely, and out in public people were really on edge. So, we walked into the pharmacy, all masked up, and I yelled at the top of my lungs: "Give us all your drugs and no one gets hurt!"

Jimmy had a heart attack thinking we'd get shot. Once they'd recovered, they appreciated my levity.

Not only is Jimmy the perfect audience for my jokes, they can give it back too!

Sometimes, as we're going out somewhere, I put on my baseball cap and sunglasses and announce performatively: "Hopefully nobody will recognize me!" But Jimmy knows me better, as does Arlene.

"You're not fooling anybody," they laugh.

Then, out in public, if I get bored, I'll just start humming loudly to turn some heads. If that doesn't work, I'll pop my cane, bounce it off the ground from one hand to another and do a box step.

After the inevitable delighted reactions from passersby, we leave and I say incredulously: "How did they recognize me?"

"Number one," Jimmy points out, laughing, "even if they don't know it's Dick Van Dyke, it's still some cool old guy dancing and singing, and who's not going to pay attention to that?!"

So now, sometimes when Jimmy sees my cane lying around, they'll start humming, pick it up, do the bounce thing and the box step, and gasp: "How did they recognize me?!"

Jimmy's got my act down pat.

CLEAR THE AIR

Most of us have our own personal strategies for cooling down threatening strangers, whether it's an irate customer at work or somebody who claims you just took their parking spot. My go-to, unsurprisingly, is comedy. There's nothing like a bit of spontaneous, self-deprecating humor to short-circuit a situation on its way to getting tense.

Now, I know from experience this tactic does not work in every situation. In the late 1950s, for instance, I found myself face-to-face with a menacing individual who proved totally immune to laughter. Be forewarned, this is a real-life horror story, but with the distance of time, I'll try my best to make it funny.

Thanks to being a morning host for CBS-TV, I received a special invitation to perform as a "guest clown" for a night with the Ringling Bros. and Barnum & Bailey Circus in Madison Square Garden. Clown at heart here! This was a dream gig!

Forgive me for not telling you much of what my actual clown duties were—you'll understand in a minute why that's not what I remember. I do recall the basics you'd expect: running goofily around in the dirt with a face full of white clown makeup.

At one point during a break in my act, I realized a) that my bladder was exploding and b) I had no idea where a bathroom was. This was the old Madison Square Garden (built in 1925), and it was a total crumbling mess. The acts with animals could enter and exit the arena through side tunnels on the ground floor, but for us lowly clowns, going "backstage" meant climbing down through a trapdoor to a dark, grim basement underneath the circus. And when I asked somebody where the men's room was, they pointed down, even lower, to another basement altogether!

After multiple descents down multiple levels and extensive wanderings through mazes of even darker, filthier and lower-ceilinged hallways, I finally found the men's room and had a good, long pee. Only afterward did I realize that I had company: a deranged-looking homeless guy standing in the corner.

The whole time I washed my hands, I could feel him looking at me. Finally, he said what was on his mind: "How do you get that stuff off?"

Oh, right! I was wearing clown makeup! No wonder he was staring!

"Well, basically just cold cream and water," I replied amiably.

This next part sounds like a movie, but trust me, it really happened.

"How about I just cut your head off instead?" he suggested with a smile.

At first, I couldn't exactly process what he had said, then he lifted up a shiny little knife to make his message loud and clear.

My heart pretty much stopped. I realized in an instant that if I were to make a break for the door, he could easily jump in my way and get some good stabbing in, even if I could wrestle past him.

This is where my instinct for tension-defusing humor kicked in. Praying that the guy was maybe not really *murder*-crazy and just having a bit of "fun" with me, I tried to go along with his "joke." Sadly, what actually came out of my mouth is forgotten, but I am sure it was a flailing attempt at humor. Knowing me, here are some distinct possibilities:

"Yes, but think of the mess! Who's gonna clean that up?!"

"Thanks, but I'll stick to cold cream and water."

"I don't think too many people will see the humor in a headless clown."

Whatever I said, it definitely didn't make him laugh. But it did at least keep him stumped long enough for me to bolt out the door, unstabbed. I sprinted down the hallway, found the stairs and was back up in the safety of my fellow performers before I could let myself breathe. My whole body was shaking and under the paint, my face was surely just as white.

I hadn't heard the guy chasing after me as I escaped, and when Garden security finally got around to looking for him, he was gone. I removed my makeup the civilized way and went straight home.

Scary part over. Exhale.

In the years since then, I've had much better luck with easing tension through humor. Of course, I've also steered clear of clown-killers.

But I have had to contend with some volatile male energy. That bird-flipper in Denver was just a drive-by, but sometimes it's been face-to-face.

Last year, Jimmy and I were taking a walk in Malibu, and a group of four men came rushing out of a store, right toward us.

"Hey! Dick Van Dyke!"

They weren't aggressive or anything, but they had a certain unsettling energy. They were boisterous. Of course, Jimmy picked up on this, and as the guys came over to say hi, Jimmy inched a little closer to me.

Because, in addition to being our assistant at home, part of Jimmy's job is security when we're out and about. As in bodyguard. Usually, they're just making sure that an excited fan doesn't accidentally topple me in one way or another.

This time was different, though, because the "stranger threat" wasn't really aimed at me.

Jimmy has a wrestler's build and can exude a lot of masculine energy in a situation like this. But at the same time, their hair was dyed a ravishing pink, shaved on the sides, and they were wearing a big NONBINARY T-shirt.

These four guys were the kind of people that couldn't just take all of that in stride. When Jimmy stepped in, they made a big deal out of being confused and offended.

"What, are you his bodyguard or something?" they said to Jimmy.

And that's as far as it got. Because luckily, I still have my magic air-clearer. Without missing a beat, I pointed my thumb at my chest and said with a big smile:

"I'm *his* bodyguard."

And it worked! Sure enough, the guys cracked up and we all shared a fun, happy moment, then Jimmy and I kept on walking. I realize now that I got Jimmy's pronouns wrong, but they cut me a lot of slack in that department. Once we were far enough away from the guys, Jimmy and I had another laugh on our own. Like: "whew."

Luckily, most of us face this kind of almost-bad situation far more often than the really bad Madison Square Garden variety. We're not bumping into killers all the time, but we do come across plenty of otherwise decent people who have, for whatever reason, let themselves get temporarily mean. Some of you might use random compliments to soothe a stranger's temper, and there are all sorts of ways to "redirect" someone when things turn dicey.

Based on my own years of experience in this arena, here are a few overall guiding principles that will come in handy, no matter which strategy you're using.

- Keep your ego out of it. Think of yourself as playing the part of a better person, even if you don't feel like one.
- Take no bait. Do not escalate.
- Smile and laugh like you mean it.
- Your mission is never to put your "adversary" down or "in their place." Your mission is to lift them up! To make them feel better!

In the end, you won't have just defused a single confrontation. You will have helped someone feel what it's like to let go of anger. And hopefully, they'll carry that feeling with them back home.

GET A SECOND OPINION (AND A THIRD AND A FOURTH . . .)

Unsolved mystery ailments: the bane of an elder's existence. Aches that pop up and worry us, for which our doctors have no useful explanation. Pain that inexplicably sharpens, visits to one bewildered specialist after another. Is it muscular? Is it neurological? Is it something serious that might be treated or fixed, or something "ordinary" that we will just have to live with? Is it all in our head?!

If only this maddening process could follow the efficient dramatic structure of a television procedural, where everything gets neatly wrapped up in one hour! In my show *Diagnosis: Murder*, for instance, each episode's mystery ended with a grand, satisfying explanation of who did the murder and how and why, grounded in cold, rational logic (except for that episode where the killer was an actual vampire).

My real-life medical mystery, meanwhile, has dragged on for almost twenty agonizing seasons, from 2006 to now. It has been full of physical misery, frustration, and despair, failed diagnoses, false hope and an overwhelming dose of convoluted scientific terminology.

To tell the truth, it's just too painful to rehash the details, and they'd probably bore you anyway. Instead I'll present the story the way I wish it had unfolded, as a mercifully brief episode of a TV mystery, complete with a whodunnit-worthy "ah-ha" climax.

THE MYSTERY: Dull ache in patient's head that sounded and felt like a heartbeat, materializing without warning in the morning and during attempted afternoon naps. Resulting in great fatigue, which diminishes the patient's capacity to work, be happy, and feel sane.

INVESTIGATION: A neuropsychiatrist friend conducts a thorough examination: medical history, blood work, brain scans and electrodes to patient's head.

DIAGNOSIS: Hypothalamus-something-or-another out of whack.

SOLUTION: Mood-and-energy-enhancing pill!

PLOT TWIST: Fatigue temporarily abated, patient peppier, but original, underlying symptoms persist and worsen.

ALL IS LOST: Patient's beloved publicist releases ill-advised dire prognosis: patient suffers from "yet-to-be diagnosed neurological disorder."

DESPERATE HAIL MARY: Patient seeks answer from Twitter. "My head bangs every time I lie down. I've had every test come back that I'm perfectly healthy. Anybody got any ideas?"

TRUE CULPRIT FINALLY REVEALED (thank you doctors who used to be on Twitter): *Titanium dental implants!*

HUMOROUS FINALE: "Well, who needs teeth?"
Roll credits.

Well, sadly, life is not TV. The implants were removed and replaced with dentures, but that infernal throbbing still lingers. The case, I'm afraid, is cold.

Will we ever find out the tooth? Stay tuned.

LEARN FROM TEACHING

In 2018, the Malibu Playhouse called up and asked for my help with a show. They're my local theater and I'd worked with them for years, so of course I would be inclined to say yes on the spot. Then, they told me it was a stage production of *Mary Poppins*, with a cast of grade schoolers, and I said: "Yes, yes, YEEEEEEEES!!"

They wanted me to be kind of an informal "guest director," sitting in on some rehearsals, giving the kids notes, talking about the movie, the play, theater in general—a breeze of a job, perfectly suited to a ninety-three-year-old guy with some pep still in his step and a five-minute commute.

Let me tell you, though, I took that job as seriously as I did my part in *Mary Poppins.* Because, in case you didn't know it by now, that's who I am. And the most important lesson I could give these kids is my abiding ethos that the stage is sacred space.

When I arrived, the kids were beside themselves with excitement. And, okay, so was I. When things died down, we talked, I told some stories from the movie, did a little singing and dancing, and then it was down to business.

I sat up front with the show's director to watch the rehearsal, pad and pen at the ready, channeling my eagle-eyed high school drama teacher Mrs. Miller. This was one of the cast's first full run-throughs in costume, so as you can imagine, I was scribbling away.

First impressions: These kids didn't need any lesson from me on taking theater seriously. They were just as committed and professional as all the child actors I'd ever worked with in movies and plays (except maybe Matthew from *Mary Poppins*). They knew their lines and they could sing and dance great. They were making the most of their costumes, and all of them brought their own idiosyncratic charm to their parts.

Now, my notes. Or rather, my brain's panicked scramble to come up with notes. Which often began with me, wondering in my seat: *What the heck are those adorable little creatures doing up there?!*

To give these kids actionable advice, I needed first to understand why they had made the choices they did. At that point in my life, I really thought I had "kid thinking" down pat! But boy, did I need a refresher.

1. WHY ARE THEY ALWAYS DROPPING CHARACTER?!

For the most part, these young actors delivered their lines with intention and emotional clarity. They put their hearts into the words and it showed on their faces.

Then, hiccup! As soon as they'd finished their lines, their faces would sag, their bodies would slouch, they'd fuss with their costume and look around while the other actors continued on with their own lines.

Then that kid would finish his lines and he'd go limp too. Over and over! When it came time for someone's next line, they'd perk right up again and deliver it perfectly, then turn off all over again.

It was like a room of buggy light bulbs! Or a lab full of briefly reanimated corpses! Or—ooooh, wait, could that really be it?

It was like a TV show!

Think, for example, of a two-person argument scene in a sitcom or soap. After one character delivers their lines on-screen, it cuts to the other character.

Of course, these kids had just learned from watching TV! After their line was done, as far as they were concerned, they were "off camera," free to invisibly fidget.

With that insight, I delivered my first note: "When you're not talking, the audience can still see you." And just as important: "Acting is reacting!"

With some regular repetition, that did the trick. All the light bulbs stayed on.

However, they didn't quite carry this first note into other aspects of their performances.

2. IS THIS GEOMETRY CLASS?

When it came to blocking, the kids had their marks figured out fine. But when they were actually on them, they'd just stand there stiffly like they'd die if they moved an inch. When they had moves, they'd drop their heads and look at their feet as they walked, in a perfectly straight line, to reach their next mark.

To figure out this problem, I again had to put myself in their shoes, then imagine their process. In earlier rehearsals, learning to "hit their mark" had required them to control their movement with uncomfortable precision. Once they'd mastered that part, they'd breathed a sigh of relief and thought their job was over.

On impulse, I leaped up and did my most exaggerated version of what they looked like to me. Which cracked them up. Followed by a gamut of more natural types of movement, on the same marks and along the same paths: crouches, flounces, stomps, hands on hips.

They got it right away. Move naturally. Movement is part of acting too.

3. I CAN'T SEE YOU AND I CAN'T HEAR YOU!

During ensemble numbers, they had a really weird habit of turning around and singing upstage. From their body language and the little I heard of their voices, they seemed to be getting into it.

But the audience was behind them. They weren't performing to us!

Well, who were they performing to?

Ohhhh, right. Each other!

Singing and dancing with each other is what kids do *naturally*. They were having their own little party up there!

Once I got them to turn downstage and sing out, I could see them get it, the power of facing the audience—even just the few of us in rehearsal—lifting their performances.

Naturally, the boy who played Bert the Chimney Sweep was a little nervous having me in the audience. But he wasn't at all trying to mimic me, and I had no notes for him in that department. His Bert was all his own.

On opening night, those kids brought it. Their self-confidence was just glowing, and I was so proud of them. Of course, a few younger kids couldn't resist the temptation to smile and wave at their parents in the crowd, but at that point, a director's job is done.

Chuckling myself to sleep that night, it occurred to me that directing kids is just like any relationship. The other person is weird. But if you don't do the work to figure their weirdness out, all you'll do is fight or talk past each other. Only once you get how their brains and hearts work can you actually communicate.

CROSS OFF REGRETS

I had a great run with movies, TV, and theater but there are so many projects and roles I had a shot at, but didn't get to do. Every now and then, one of these almosts will pop into my brain and I'll slap my forehead.

When producers were adapting the musical *Oliver!* for film, they offered me the part of Fagin, the criminal mastermind of a band of pickpocketing kids. But early in rehearsals, there was a behind-the-scenes disagreement that I won't get into, and I dropped out. That choice still stings me.

One day, my agent got a call from Sophia Loren's manager, who said that Sophia would like to do a comedy with me. My agent said no on the spot and only told me about it later.

"What?!" I hollered.

The money was no good, my agent said, and I would have had to take second billing. I told him I didn't care if they didn't mention my name at all! I would have paid to be in a movie with Sophia Loren! In all her movies I'd seen, she was pure electricity, up for all sorts of risk-taking and wildly funny. We would have had a blast together!

But it was too late. This one hurts a little differently, because I don't even know what the movie was!

Once I was offered a part in a New York revival of *Who's Afraid of Virginia Woolf?*, playing George, the miserably acerbic college professor who trades vicious barbs with his wife Martha for hours and hours. I know I could have brought the comedy to that role.

But again, my agent turned the role down without even asking me! Note to agents: Do not ever do this.

The legendary mime Marcel Marceau was my idol. When he was working down in Greenwich Village, I made every single Wednesday matinee. I finally got a backstage pass to go meet him, and much to my surprise, the man famous for silence turned into a regular Henny Youngman! Cracking one-liners left and right.

Much, much later, in the early 2000s, both Marcel and I agreed to come out of our non-retirements and work together on a television special—with mime performance as its centerpiece. What a dream and honor! To do mime alongside this great!

For a time, it felt like the project was really coming together. But then, at the peak of my excitement, I got terrible news: my dear Marcel had died. It was heartbreaking.

Even now, though, I can conjure our show perfectly in my mind, which helps soften the regret.

There's one "almost" that I've gone back and forth on for years. Believe it or not, I was up for a part in *The Omen*—the father of Damien the devil boy. This was the post-*Exorcist* 1970s and Hollywood was all in on evil little kids. I guess the producers were looking for someone more likable for the father role, maybe to give the film a moral center.

I read the script (though I've blocked out the details) and concluded that the death and gore were just way too much.

This was not fun horror, this was *disturbing*. After I turned the role down, the producers found someone even squeakier clean than me: Atticus Finch, aka Gregory Peck.

In a 2013 interview with *The Telegraph*, I expressed regret over my decision: "My God, that was stupid . . . I was pretty puritan at the time, a Goody Two-shoes . . . I felt I'd put myself in a position where the audience trusted me."

Well, twelve years later, I've changed my mind again. Arlene just looked up *The Omen* to fill me in on the details of the script I had blocked out. A lightning rod impales a priest, a devil dog makes a nanny hang herself at a kid's birthday party, somebody is decapitated, and my would-have-been character tries to stab Damien in the skull on a church altar with some special knives.

Call me a Goody Two-shoes, but I now stand by my original decision. At least that's one regret I can cross off the list.

LEARN FROM SHAME

It starts just like an episode of *The Dick Van Dyke Show*. I am on the couch in the living room, smoking. Mary walks in and wonders why I'm in such a good mood.

"I have the two things that would make any man happy," I reply. "A gorgeous wife. And a Kent."

"Which do you like best?" she asks.

"Now there's a tough one," I reply, earning chuckles from the audience. After some deliberation, I conclude that I like my wife better for her dancing, kissing, and cooking, and my cigarette better for its "filter and taste."

"I'll accept that," says Mary, lighting up a Kent of her own.

As soon as the ad aired, Mary and I both felt total horror. *What did we just do?!*

We had put our names and images, and our show's image, on an ad for cigarettes! This was our first season, so we were more beholden to our sponsors, for sure.

But this was 1961, not 1940. And by then, everybody knew the medical truth about smoking, even if the tobacco companies wouldn't admit it: cigarettes were addictive and dangerous. Both Mary and I were heavy smokers at the time and regularly trying to quit, so we knew this personally.

However belatedly, we listened to our consciences and took action. We told Carl and our agents, who told the network and Kent, that we'd made a grave error in judgment and we wanted the spot killed as quickly as was contractually possible.

After that first time, it never aired again.

Lesson learned. We were celebrities now and that came with responsibility. After that, Mary and I took that responsibility very seriously.

The raw footage for that Kent ad still exists online. For me, it's kind of a jabbing reminder that some regrets can't be just crossed off, that certain mistakes will follow you forever.

NEVER CALL "CUT"

When I heard they were doing a new *Mary Poppins* movie, I said: "Can I be in it?!"

They gave me a knockout of a cameo right at the end. I played Mr. Dawes Jr., the ninety-year-old son of the ninety-year-old banker I'd played in the first movie. Which was handy: I'd grown into the part, no more elaborate aging necessary.

Then, when it came time for hair and makeup, I sat in that chair forever. They gave me a white mustache, a wig, and mutton chops, everything. I said: "Do you guys realize you're doing all this work to make a ninety-two-year-old guy look like a ninety-year-old guy?"

We had two days to film my big scene, and it was a real celebration of elder empowerment. Mr. Dawes Jr. has been shoved aside in the family banking business by his scheming nephew (Colin Firth), derided as a doddering, senile "loony." He is anything but.

First, I got to dress down Colin Firth. Then I got to prove him wrong with a little song and dance.

When they've told you that you're finished and your
chance to dance is done

That's the time to stand, to strike up the band, and tell them you've just begun.

From there, it was on to filming my climactic moment: I would cast my cane aside, do a lithe high-step prance across the office, then climb up onto the bank president's desk and tap-dance! Quite a feat for a ninety-two-year-old, which was precisely the point of the scene.

Director Rob Marshall had some concerns that I'd be able to pull it off, and frankly, so did I—especially getting up onto that desk without wiping out, much less looking graceful.

So, to aid in my ascent, Rob had a chair placed in front of the desk, then a stool a bit farther back, so I could stairstep my ascent. And, in case I lost my balance, Lin-Manuel Miranda would be standing by in the scene to give me a discreet hand.

Safety precautions in place, Rob called "action!" Discard cane—perfect! Cross-office prance—hilarious and so very me! And now, the hard part . . .

Big step up! Right over the stool, not even touching it, bouncing up from the chair . . .

Big step 2—onto the desk, perfect landing!!!

And "cut!"

The mood on the set, Arlene recalls, was "wow," from Lin, Rob, Emily Blunt (as Mary Poppins), and the rest of the cast and crew. A bit winded, I stood on the desk and took it in.

Then, after a huddle with the crew, Rob announced we needed another take—nothing to do with my performance, rest assured, that's just the way it goes with movies. There were plenty of worried looks all around—can Dick do it again?!—but I dismounted that desk and returned to my starting spot like a pro.

Take 2: just as great! Print!

Then came a new camera setup for my real fun: the desktop dance. Tapping, finger-snapping, hip wiggles, and finally, outright swaggery stomping. I loved every step!

When I wrapped up the dance, I saw everybody just beaming. Later, Emily said that she was in tears. The first and last time I've made anyone cry with a tap dance.

Believe it or not, that wasn't the climax of the scene. Pooped from his dancing, Dawes slumps into his chair, retakes his rightful place as head of the bank, and delivers a monologue that calls back to a scene from the original *Mary Poppins*, assuring that the desperate Banks family will keep their beloved home from bank seizure, and the film will have its happy ending.

I performed that speech with all my heart. When I was done, there was a very long, pregnant silence. That went on . . . and on . . . and on. I never broke character, of course. But finally, off camera, heads started turning to Rob.

He stood there motionless, his mouth a little open, so overwhelmed with emotion that he couldn't call "cut." Which was just how the rest of us felt too.

DON'T MATCH JIMMY

At ninety-nine years old, I still try to hit the gym three times a week. I don't know why this is something I still want to do, but it is. I'm not a "wake up and go back to bed" type just yet, unless it's cold and rainy.

If I miss too many gym days, I really can feel it—a stiffness creeping in here and there in my joints. If I let that set in, well, God help me. When I'm sluggish and reluctant, here are some of the "carrots" I dangle in front of myself to get out the door:

- huge smoothie and/or frothy caffeine treat after my workout
- full-body tingly exhilaration
- sharper mind
- sense of accomplishment to bask in for the rest of the day
- naptime, well-earned
- limber dancing in the days ahead

At the gym, I usually do a circuit, going from one machine to the next without a break, in a circle. I start with sit-ups on the sit-up machine. Arlene says I could do five hundred, but that might be exaggerating. Then it's lower body—I do all the leg machines religiously and repeatedly because my legs are two of my most cherished possessions. And then the upper body.

The secret ingredient to my gym time is the music. For some reason, our gym is sparsely attended in the early mornings—bad for the owners, but perfect for me and Arlene. She knows how to get into their sound system, so she always brings my kind of stuff, and she really blasts it. The place has great acoustics, which is not something you can say for most gyms.

And it's the music that really gets me going.

Starting position. Me-me-me-me!

Exhale into the lift, or the push, or the pull . . . and hum into it!

Peak contraction (if I'm lucky): break briefly into song!

Return and inhale.

Next set, next verse!

To be honest, most of my humming and singing really happens when I'm between sets, going from one machine to another. By "going," I mean dancing. You heard me, dancing! A little soft-shoe, maybe a kick or a shimmy, whatever little show the song brings out in me. And if I'm really feeling it, I'm no quiet warbler; I'm a Broadway belter.

By the end of my workout, I'm in a sweaty rush, the blood flowing fingertips to toes, and my spirits are soaring.

Okay, today, what's next?!

Often, Jimmy comes with us to the gym and works out too, but their routine is different: the standard three sets on one muscle, then on to another. Usually, Jimmy is lifting pretty heavy weights, which is quite impressive.

Every now and then, I like a little challenge, and Jimmy will catch me increasing my weight on a machine to what they were doing.

One time, I got even bolder, up for a fresh challenge. Maybe, I'll admit, feeling a bit competitive. Jimmy hopped off one machine, and then I slipped on, keeping the weight the same.

Oh my God that's heavy. But I—can—do—it!

Next machine they hopped off, I was right there.

One machine after another, I followed Jimmy's whole circuit! Sure, I was rubbery all over, but also thoroughly exhilarated!

Afterward, I swaggered over to Jimmy and announced: "I've been matching you."

Jimmy seemed unsurprised, so I guess they'd been watching me the whole time. "Are you sure you want to do that?"

A reasonable question. Jimmy is a forty-one-year-old athlete. I am ninety-nine.

"Yeah, I just wanted to see what I can do."

The next day, Jimmy came to work, and I was sore and hobbling.

"That was a bad idea," I admitted.

DON'T LIVE IN THE PAST

I do like to reminisce on occasion (e.g., reruns with Carl, writing this book), but I don't want to live there. And there's a real difference between the two.

When Margie and I were first married, we rented a little one-room guesthouse way up Laurel Canyon. The main house was owned by a retired actress who I'd never heard of. Every night, she'd start drinking, then stumble down to our place and start telling us stories about her life in the theater.

She drove us nuts. Here we were, starting a fresh life, me diving into a new career, and all her stories sucked the energy right out of us.

These days, I find the same thing happens when I'm around another old person. They just want to tell stories about stuff that's already happened a long time ago.

At a recent public event, I forget what it was, an old producer came over through the crowd to say hello. I didn't know him at all when we both had Hollywood careers, but I guarantee you this: whenever there are two old guys together out in public, everybody assumes they're best friends, they'll just naturally have something to talk about, and it will make a great picture.

So, as we're standing there with the cameras flashing, he starts telling me all these stories about people way back when that we may have had in common, reliving his old memories that I wasn't even really a part of. If this was Carl, and we had more in common, I wouldn't have been so itchy.

He's a really warmhearted guy, and I smiled along with it for a while. But then my eyes glazed over. I felt terrible, but I wasn't able to absorb a word he was saying!

Arlene clocked all of this and came over to the rescue, getting me out of there as soon as was politely possible. Coming to my senses, I groused unkindly: "All he talks about is the past."

The fact is: nobody wants to hear old people running on. Including me. Especially about stuff that doesn't matter anymore.

At least let's talk about the present, if not the future!

For me, the "eyes glazing over" is a good internal barometer, whether it's somebody else dwelling too much on bygones or me doing it myself. If I feel energy seeping out of my voice or my brain going slack, that's a telltale sign that I'm lapsing too deep into memory land. Then, if I'm not careful, it will feel like a scrim coming down between me and the actual world around me, getting more and more opaque. (I'm sure that old actress would appreciate my theater metaphor!)

Wake up, Dick! What and who are right in front of you, right now?! Grab on, jump in! As soon as I start to feel a sense of quickening, that's my lifeline back to the present.

And as for the future, here's a little internal checklist I keep handy: What are you going to do today? What do you want tomorrow, next month, next year to look like? What feels important? What still needs getting done?

The opposites of "glazed over" are sharp, urgent, and alive. Don't those feel so much better?

IT PAYS TO GO TO THE GYM

In 1965, *The Dick Van Dyke Show* was reaching the end of its run on CBS. Meanwhile, flip the channel over to NBC during the afternoon, and a very different show was just getting started: *Days of Our Lives*, which is still going strong in its sixtieth year.

It's fitting then, since I too am going strong, that I'd make my daytime debut on that show at the age of ninety-seven. Though I can't say I saw it coming. Like it had so many other times in my life, a door opened and I just walked through it.

It all started at my gym. My workout there often overlapped with another actor, Drake Hogestyn, who'd been a star of *Days of Our Lives* since 1986. Drake's character John and Deirdre Hall's Marlena were one of the show's longest running love stories, and together they'd survived serial killers, kidnappings, identity switch-ups, amnesia, and repeated satanic possessions.

Now most of that I learned secondhand. I've never kept up with daytime soap operas, mainly because I've rarely been in front of a TV at the same time, five days a week. Also, the pace is a little too slow for me.

But every now and then, between sets at the gym, I would give Drake a little half rib/half pitch: "Don't they ever hire any old people on that show? Come on!"

Unbeknownst to me, Drake took me seriously, talked to the show's producers and suddenly, they had a special guest part for me with a four-episode storyline!

My part was a "John Doe," an old war vet who shows up at the hospital with no memory of his entire life. (Ironically, when I recently told the story of my character, I forgot I'd played an amnesiac and Arlene had to remind me!) Slowly but surely, the kind "Doc" Marlena helps me unlock my memories, and in a classic soap opera twist, I realize I am the long-lost father of Drake's character John, who, heretofore has been searching for me in vain.

Arlene even got a part, as Officer Silver, the cop who first pushes me in in a wheelchair. She'd never acted professionally before and was in a panic that she'd blow the scene. I helped her with her lines and gave her some pointers, and she nailed it.

As we did our shooting, one thing struck me as odd: it's so quiet on those soap opera sets. The actors have all been doing it for so many years, they just come in and do their lines and that's that—all business. It's certainly a secure way to make a living, but I would imagine it gets awfully dull.

Well, I tried to pep things up a little bit while I was there. I made jokes with my castmates as much as I could, doing my silly rendition of the soap opera cliffhanger music. One time, during a very serious scene, I accidentally cracked myself up and we had to do another take. Which the soaps don't at all like to do. And they even let me throw in some trademark singing and soft-shoe with two of the oldest cast members, Bill Hayes and Susan Seaforth Hayes.

Now, I'm hardwired for comedy, so I didn't take naturally to the beats of that kind of drama. Plus, at the beginning of practically every other scene of a soap, the characters do a little recap of what came before, in case the audience missed it or something. With my bad memory, I was already prone to repeating myself, so this was hilariously disconcerting.

"Wait," I'd say, perusing a new day's script. "Didn't I say this yesterday?"

One day, they threw me for a real loop, giving me a script for scenes that I hadn't prepared for yet. Apparently, I'd been given the script for the following day by mistake. "Give me thirty minutes," I said like a real pro, and memorized it on the spot.

I guess I wasn't half bad as an old amnesiac—I won a Daytime Emmy! In my acceptance speech, I joked that "I feel like a spy from nighttime television." The truth is I felt like I'd been welcomed into a family.

Sadly, I lost two of my *Days* scene partners less than a year after shooting—Bill Hayes who was ninety-eight, and my rock-solid gym buddy and on-screen son, Drake Hogestyn, who lost his battle to pancreatic cancer at age seventy.

In the wake of their deaths, there was an outpouring of grief from fans of the show, who'd grown up with these characters and felt deeply connected and loyal. That's another thing I learned about soaps as a spy from nighttime TV: the audience is part of the family too.

BUILD A SLIDE AND GRANDKIDS WILL COME

Having established that play is the secret to life, and that children are the original owners of that secret, our duty as adults becomes clear: to do anything and everything we can to keep kids playing. For inspiration in this effort, I invite you to look out my living room window.

Whenever my many grandkids or great-grandkids come over, the backyard and pool are where the action is. And Arlene and I are always dreaming up new ways to make the place feel like Adventure Land.

Before she moved in, the whole hillside back there was just a brushy blank, wasted space. Arlene cleared it all out, created railroad-tie terraces and windy stone paths and steps, and everywhere, there's a constantly evolving show of native California plants and wildflowers. We also put in a bunch of little outbuildings (which we call "she-sheds"), all at different levels on the hillside, each with its own special path and stairs. The whole place looks like a lush magical hobbit paradise, perfect for grandkids and great-grandkids to play, to sneak around and get "lost," to spin out adventures.

Of course, like any grandparent or great-grandparent, I wish they'd visit more often. Just hearing them all out there squealing gives me such joy.

A few years ago, I hit on a new plan to entice them over: I had a custom waterslide built in the pool. The slide looks a little like something out of *The Swiss Family Robinson*, if *The Swiss Family Robinson* had a cement mixer. It's a long, steep concrete trough clad in a jumble of rough-hewn stones.

On opening day, it took exactly three seconds to declare the new attraction a success. One great-grandkid shot down that thing and skidded into the pool, then another and another. The adults waited their turns and screamed all the way down, just like the kids. If the kids were too scared or little, my grandson Shane or another adult would hold them tight and ride down with them. We had four generations going down that thing, all afternoon.

It's a steep climb up the stairs to the launching pad at the top of the slide, but that didn't slow them down.

"Again!" "Again!" "Again!"

By the end of the day, everybody's hindquarters were raw, but they didn't feel it until the next morning. At Barry's house, they all woke up with sore butts and wondered: *What the hell is this?* A couple of times going down, you don't feel it. But it's rough enough that a hundred times, your epidermis is going to pay the price.

Now that the slide is old hat, I'm scheming again. Behind and above the pool, there's kind of a blank spot on the hill that I have my eye on. Arlene is picturing a little train. I'm thinking rope swing, though maybe that'd be too dangerous. What about a zip line? That area is just begging for some kind of new ride.

TRANSMOGRIFY HALLOWEEN (ON FAMILY TRADITIONS)

I was tinkering out in our garage in Encino one day during the 1960s, and a little boy from down the street came over and asked me what I was doing.

"I'm making a monster," I told him, and his eyes went wide.

For me, my wife Margie, and our four kids, Halloween was fast becoming our favorite family tradition. Eclipsing Christmas and the Fourth of July by a mile.

I know the roots of my own obsession with "playing scary": Boris Karloff and my little graveyard school play. As an actor, transformation is kind of your lifeblood, and it's what Halloween is all about too. When I became a parent, I passed this love on to my children too. Margie and I encouraged them to run wild with their imaginations, to dream up whoever or whatever they wanted to be, and we put weeks into their masterpieces every year. I must admit, I was probably more excited about the costume-*making* part than they were.

Out of that simple joy, the rest of our Halloween blossomed, and once we moved to Encino, it really had room to grow. We had a huge front yard with a half-circle driveway, a garden with a pond in front, all underneath these big oak trees—a landscape perfect for turning into a haunted wildland. Each year, we welcomed the whole neighborhood in to brave our creations: bats, witches, and ghouls dangling in the branches; mummies in the underbrush; a creature in the black lagoon.

I had tried my hand at Frankenstein's Monster before, but this year, I was really going wild with it.

Once that little neighbor boy found out what I was doing, he was at my side every day, watching my progress. I molded and sculpted a huge head, a perfect Boris Karloff, let it set and painted the hair and the green face.

Then I made the body. I set the form up on a big table and used an erector set inside the chest to go up and down so the thing would look like it was breathing. I recorded myself doing this deep monster growly breathing, in and out, put the tape on a loop and hid the player in the chest. I timed the thing perfectly so the inhale-exhale was in sync with the chest going up and down. It was a pretty good illusion for homemade.

Every day, that kid's eyes got bigger and bigger. He was seeing the whole thing come together, all the mechanics, inside and out.

Once I finally finished it, I had him step back a little to get a good view. Then, I turned on a blue light shining down on it and started up the breathing.

Suddenly, that kid was screaming his head off and ran home as fast as he could. It didn't matter that he knew it was fake, that he'd seen how it was made. Now it was a real monster!

Once it came time for the public unveiling of my Boris, I'm pretty sure that kid would not set foot on our property. Eventually, he got brave enough to come over to the house, but never to the basement, where he knew the monster was stored.

Over the years, our Encino Halloween got more elaborate. I brought a special effects crew in from Disney to light the whole thing, blast a fog machine, add crazy sound effects and creatures that actually moved.

Later, with my partner Michelle in our Malibu home, the escalation of Dick Van Dyke's Halloween Extravaganza continued. By the time I married Arlene, I had movie-grade special effects and equipment trucks down the block. It was like something you'd find at an amusement park, and I don't mean rickety old Coney Island, I mean Universal Studios.

The first year, I thought Arlene loved it. The second year, I noticed something was amiss. In the middle of our big street party, I couldn't find her anywhere. I was pretty sure I'd seen her getting into an Elvira costume?

I ventured back inside and through the house, and there she was, by herself in our empty backyard.

What is the Mistress of the Night doing back here all alone? I thought my new wife adored Halloween! Wasn't that one of the big things we had in common?

"It's too big," Arlene told me, and then she unloaded. "It's like a movie set. It's just this whole other world that is foreign to me and I don't know where I fit. It's not me."

Well, that sure sunk my Halloween spirit. But I got what Arlene was saying right away. This was my thing, not ours.

So, after that Halloween, we decided together to throw in the towel on the over-the-top Halloween and sold most of the stuff off to our neighbor James Cameron.

Well, the next year, Arlene went over to his Halloween and loved it, but then she came home to our empty little house and felt horrible. Not having any Halloween at all felt wrong.

Out of the ashes sprung Dick and Arlene Van Dyke's New Halloween, officially known as Vandy Manor. A party on a much more manageable scale, a tradition we both could invent together.

The vision was simple: less block-long theme park, more backyard costume party. Everybody dresses up, we do good old-fashioned trick-or-treating, maybe a little live show, and of course, scaring and spooking and squealing. But from humans, not machines.

For our first year, Arlene was Ursula, the purple sea witch from *The Little Mermaid*. Which involved a lot of purple body paint and looked amazing. But Arlene didn't just want to be Ursula, she wanted to do Ursula. So, she learned every line of Ursula's blockbuster number, "Poor Unfortunate Souls," so she could lip-synch it perfectly.

Regrettably, my wardrobe choice wasn't quite as fun.

The plan was for me to be Arlene's warm-up act, doing a kind of spoken-word version of "Thriller." And I thought my costume was just as perfect as hers. It was a brown robe and a creepy old lady mask I'd cut the bottom out of, which turned my face into some gruesome, pieced-together mutant—half hag, half Dick.

Just one step into the spotlight for my big debut, and suddenly, kids started screeching, running behind their parents' legs or out into the street. I had no idea what was going on and immediately forgot all the words to the song. Then the parents scooped the kids up and they all started crying together, faces buried in their parents' chests, afraid to open their eyes, much less look my way. It was a huge mess.

What happened?! I felt so guilty and confused. In past years, my costumes had scared kids plenty—but in a gleeful way, the way kids love to be scared! This year, it was entirely different. I had frightened these kids out of their wits, just like I'd terrified that kid in Encino with my breathing Boris Karloff! Once things died down, I slunk into the bathroom, took a good hard look in the mirror and realized that yes, Dick, this year, you've taken things too far.

I'm afraid I eclipsed Ursula.

But on our next Halloween and all the Halloweens since, Ursula has become not just part of the show, but the star. She does that number with all the sinister, campy bombast of the cartoon original, complete with Cruella cackle as she steals poor Ariel's voice.

Among our regular young guests, she is now legendary. A neighbor tells us that every time she and her daughter walk by our house, her daughter says excitedly: "Do you know who lives here?" Of course, you'd think she might be referring to Bert or Mr. Chitty Bang Bang.

"The sea witch lives here!" she says.

Meanwhile, our Halloween has ballooned into gigantic again, now with Arlene's full buy-in—the backyard *and* the street, with all the bells and whistles. Having scared those kids witless, however, I lost my enthusiasm for dressing up. One year, Arlene got me a scarecrow costume, since I love *The Wizard of Oz*, but I wouldn't commit to the hair or makeup. "You look like you're in your pajamas," she complained.

Eventually, I got a much-needed education in properly scaring children. Jimmy and their partner Robin became part of the show, and boy were they good. One year, after sending a gaggle of adults and kids shrieking down the street, they came back inside for a break, and I exclaimed proudly: "You scared the shit out of them!" The first time they'd heard me curse.

Observing them more closely one night, I realized there was careful strategy at work. They only went for little kids if there were parents in tow who looked game. Regardless of age, they got a bead on how much "scary" their audience or victim could take, and modulated accordingly.

Inspired, I donned a simple little zombie-like mask and went outside later that night. The younger kids were all gone and the teenagers were creeping in, which we all know means nothing but mischief. I positioned myself in among a little group of identical zombie mannequins and stood frozen there, awaiting my prey.

Those boys came swaggering over and started pushing and squeezing on all the mannequins, sneering at how they weren't scary. One kid got to me and started poking . . .

And suddenly, I came alive and grabbed his wrist!

He jerked away in terror and yelped: "Mama!"

Finally, after all these years, a scare I can be proud of.

THE CLOTHES MAKE THE GNOME

Producers of *The Masked Singer* had been trying to get me on their show for years, but Arlene always turned them down. The whole thing just weirded us out.

Here's the show's basic premise: Celebrities of all sorts, singers and non-singers alike, get hidden in these absurdly elaborate creature costumes, then perform songs for a live audience and a panel of judges, who try to guess who they are based on their singing voices and some biographical clues.

Gladys Knight was a steampunk bee. The three Brady boys were mummies. According to Arlene, Johnny Rotten of the Sex Pistols (don't ask me who that is) wore a horned, tartaned "jester" outfit that could have spawned a horror franchise, singing a plaintive American folk tune from 1913.

When it comes time for the characters to remove their costumes and reveal their true identities, the whole audience chants: "Take it off! Take it off!" like it's a game of strip poker.

The Masked Singer, as Arlene put it, "felt like the end of the world."

Finally, in 2023, the producers offered so much money that we couldn't say no.

But Arlene did have some stipulations. First, as a ninety-seven-year-old, I needed a costume that wouldn't trip me up or suffocate me. There was also my dignity to consider. Arlene insisted that, whatever the costume was, I needed to be able to look positively dashing when I finally emerged from it as my real self. We'd seen poor William Shatner, wriggling out his Knight on a Golden Duck getup, beet red and sopping with sweat.

And when they said they wanted me to sing some contemporary pop hit, Arlene rolled her eyes and said absolutely not. I'd be doing something age and genre appropriate. I love Arlene.

When Arlene, Jimmy, and I arrived at the taping, things got strange fast. Somebody threw a sack over my head. No one, not even the crew, could know who I was. Then, they made Arlene, Jimmy, and me all put on masks, gloves, and black zippy sweatshirts that said: DON'T TALK TO ME. Which Jimmy still has and comes in handy when they're not feeling social.

Ushered backstage, we finally got to see my costume, aka my prison. My first impression was "pumpkin," but then I looked closer. And this is when my experience on *The Masked Singer* did a total one-eighty.

In all my movie roles, when I get into costume, a whole new part of the character comes alive for me. The clothes make the man, they say, and in my case as a performer, it's totally true. What I wear becomes who I am.

Turns out, my costume was not a pumpkin. It was a giant gnome. And objectively speaking, the thing was spectacular. A floor-length ginger beard with braids, a mossy-grassy cape replete with flowers and squirrels, a toadstool and little gnome house sprouting out of its cap, giant pointy ears, bedazzled headset, and comically inert gnome eyes. This was pure artistry! Those costume designers definitely loved their job.

And that love leaped right out of the gnome and into my heart. Now I wouldn't just be singing a song as me. My voice had a character to work with!

Then it came time to get me into the thing, which did kind of mute my thrill. I had a little cavity inside, which was roomy enough, but when they put all the pieces of the gnome's exterior together around me, it got really dark. There was a little screen in front that I could see out of, sort of, but no doubt about it, I was claustrophobic.

As I adjusted to my new habitat, I just kept thinking how full of love and texture Gnome looked on the outside. I wanted my voice to match that, to be that beautiful. And that's what I focused on in the dark.

Meanwhile, as shooting started, Jimmy was spiraling into a panic, unbeknownst to me or Arlene. Producers and crew members kept pulling them aside and saying: "Well if Dick goes on to the next round, that round is going to be an all-ABBA theme for all the contestants, so Dick's going to have to learn an ABBA song."

Dick Van Dyke? ABBA?!

At last, it was showtime. Gnome rolls out onstage to lots of *ooh*s and *aah*s from the crowd—did I mention that my whole costume was on wheels? For the most part, I remained on my mark, using some levers inside my costume to operate my mittened "hands" every now and then, which I hoped was a nice Gnomey touch.

My song was the classic "When You're Smiling," a joyful number that practically all the greats have recorded. I channeled Gnome and went at it with all my crooner gusto. I let the age in my voice shine, and put warmth, playfulness, and love into every lyric. From my dark interior, it sure sounded and felt like the audience was getting into it.

Behind me and around me, a big-budget Disney-colored song-and-dance unfolded with backup singers and dancers with fluffy umbrellas, a constant shower of confetti and finally a balloon drop.

Roaring applause, and according to Arlene and Jimmy, who were in the audience, a standing ovation! Still in disguise, I stood there for the judges' reactions and guesses, and Nicole Scherzinger gushed: "Your vocals melted my heart."

The other judges guessed I was Dustin Hoffman, Robert De Niro, or Tony Bennett—not bad! But when it came time for votes, Gnome came up short and was voted off—sadly or luckily, depending on how you look at it. At least now, Jimmy could breathe a sigh of relief about me doing ABBA.

Gnome's big "take it off" reveal was just as drawn-out as it looks on TV; it took some stagehands to dismantle that thing and extract me from it. When I finally appeared, I was at my most unruffled and dapper—gray plaid suit, black shirt, perfect hair, and makeup.

The whole place exploded—screaming, sobbing, cheering, bowing, judge Ken Jeong standing on the table, all of it. It filled my heart with such warmth and gratitude. The most touching of all was seeing Nicole Scherzinger and Jenny McCarthy weeping. I took a half step from my spot toward Nicole, wanting to give her a hug. "The whole world loves you so much," she said.

For an encore, I led the crowd in a rousing "Supercalifragilisticexpialidocious," which brought everybody back to their childhoods. I even threw in a bit of Bert's "Step in Time" footwork, which earned much over-the-top disbelief from the panel and panic from Arlene and Jimmy, who knew how slippery that stage floor was.

On the way home, all three of us were still buzzing. Hands down, that show was the most bizarre performance of my life—so much over-the-top pageantry! But you take all the balloons out of it, and the overflow of love on that soundstage was very real.

I owe much of my success to wardrobe. The thing I'd dreaded the most ended up being my best friend.

The Masked Singer, I stand humbly corrected.

Sincerely, Gnome.

PS: Can I keep my costume?

STAY TALL INSIDE

Recently, I realized that I have shrunk.

I used to be six foot one, and now I'm five foot nine. That's four entire inches. Where did it go?

I don't know! It hasn't happened to anyone else I know.

Probably too many pratfalls.

I've had to cut the hems of my pants off!

Am I still shrinking or am I done?

If you've been around me in the past few years, you've likely heard multiple versions of this shrinking bit. But it's not just me trying to get a laugh; it's coming from a very real place.

On the rational side, Arlene patiently reminds me that shrinking is a natural part of aging. She chides me for acting like I'm the only one this happens to.

But I just can't get over my astonishment at the sheer scale of my physical transformation over these past few years. The skinnier part I don't mind so much; Arlene admires my eight-pack.

It's the height thing that's just so weird. I guess it must have started happening a while ago, gradually. But to me it felt like somebody just took an axe to my legs last night! *Hack, hack, now you're an elf!*

To go from being a tall person, with all that tall-person gravitas, to being the shortest one in the room that people need to stoop over a little to say hello to—it's disconcerting. Am I shrinking my way out of the world? Maybe I'm fixating on getting short so much, like it's this rare "condition" happening only to me, so that I can still *feel* tall—and young—at my core.

Whatever it's about, I'm lucky to always have a rotating audience to keep the bit fresh.

My son Barry came over for coffee the other day and I asked: "Have you shrunk any?"

"Oh yeah, Mary [his wife] and I both shrunk, like about an inch and a half." Then, not missing a beat: "But we're doing it at the same rate, so it doesn't matter. I still look taller."

On another day last week, The Vantastix were here for a rehearsal. Twenty-five years ago when we started, we were pretty much the same height; now I'm the short one by a mile. Midway through the practice, we took a break.

"I've shrunk four inches since we started singing," I said.

"In an hour?" one of the guys joked.

I gave a little extra bass to my laugh and felt six one all over again.

HAND OVER THE KEYS

I love cars and I love driving—in that, I am fully Californian. For years, I was a Jaguar guy, up until the one that burned. Long before that, I had another Jag that I drove too fast and slammed into a concrete wall—I was fine, but the car wasn't.

At the height of my career, Jaguars made me feel edgier than my nice-guy persona—effortlessly cool, sexy, daring. Before the Jags, it had been all clunkers and station wagons, tools I needed to get me places. With Jaguars, I fell in love with driving for the fun of it.

I loved the usual things one loves about driving: speed, adventure, wind, freedom. Moving out to Malibu in the 1980s, I had easy access to all that: a leisurely oceanside cruise up the Pacific Coast Highway; up Tuna, Latigo, or Encinal Canyon for my own personal Le Mans.

All of which is to say that driving felt pretty central to my sense of self. So, when you hear this story, you'll know what's at stake. Every old person must face the question of "when to hand over the keys," and it can spark real crisis and grief. Some people work through this gracefully, and others, well . . .

First, let's get that final Jaguar out of the way, because that's really act one of this story.

The "minor repairs" you've heard about were not as innocuous as I made them sound. Oftentimes, when I was parking or backing up or whatever, I tended to bump and rub the car against various things. Sometimes I noticed and sometimes I didn't. It was never anything big, except for one time where it looked like somebody had punched in the trunk. I've told you I'm messy.

Well, Arlene had been noticing all these little dents and scrapes as they happened, of course. But rather than get them fixed one-by-one, she wisely waited until I had accumulated maybe five or six of them before sending the car in for repairs. So, when I got the Jaguar back just before it burned, it did indeed *look* brand-new, but the fixes were hiding my shameful secret.

A secret that continued to expose itself on the bodies of my future cars, a secret I continued to avoid. By my early nineties, I was rubbing up on other cars, and not knowing it, a lot. Arlene would park her car as far away from mine as possible, so at least we'd have one vehicle intact. Eventually, it got to a point where she really didn't want me to drive it at all.

Superficially, I gave in. Fine, I said, I'll allow you to drive us everywhere in your car. But no way was I giving up my own car, nor the idea that I could still take it for a spin anytime I pleased. Driving was *me*, remember? How could I give up me?

No surprise then, that when it came time to renew my driver's license, going to the DMV was priority number one. And guess what? I passed with flying colors, even the vision test! Which, unfortunately, reinforced my false confidence.

Act two: The past is never really dead.

On the renewal form, I filled in my correct birth year, 1925. Uh-oh, wait a second. On every official form I've ever had since I was a child, my birth date has been 1926.

Suddenly, a near-century old family secret reared its ugly head. To make a long story short (the details are in my memoir), I had been conceived before my parents were married. Out of shame, my mother had wanted to cover it up, so she changed my birth date to a year later. Now, I'd known about this lie since my grandmother revealed it to me when I was a teenager. Since then, it had never really come up, except as a funny story about my past.

But now the DMV was faced with a clear discrepancy and the whole matter would have to be looked into before I could get my new license. Then COVID hit and shut everything down, and the problem never got resolved. So, while I had the state's official endorsement of my ability to drive, I lacked the little card to prove it.

I like to think of myself as a law-abiding citizen, so this technicality did keep me from getting behind the wheel. For the most part.

But sometimes, very rarely, the injustice chafed at me, and I stood up to fight this slow surrender. Little errands, here and there, to keep what was left of my pride.

Act three opens on a very rainy day in March 2023. Claustrophobia, ants in the pants, whatever you want to call it: For some reason, I decided that I needed an immediate day-of appointment at the optometrist. Usually, Arlene or Jimmy would drive me to these kinds of things, but the rain was delaying Jimmy's commute over from Burbank, and I was pretty sure Arlene was busy with something else.

So, in my youthful, can-do mind, it made perfect sense to drive myself. The optometrist was literally just down our one little road, about a quarter mile away in the shopping plaza. What could possibly happen? I reasoned, driving the Lexus into the storm without even telling Arlene I'd gone.

That damn rain. It didn't used to rain this much in March in Southern California. But for the past several years, it's just been downpour after downpour. I got to the one-lane bridge over Malibu Creek, and it was flooded over and closed. So, I turned around and went the other way out of our community, which would involve a brief foray onto the Pacific Coast Highway, not something I looked forward to.

But before I could even make it that far, a big oncoming truck veered into my path and ran me off the road. I swerved and promptly slammed into someone's metal front fence. Thanks to the nonfunctioning airbags, my face hit the steering wheel. I tasted blood right away.

Luckily, my injuries ended up being very minor: a few cuts, one of which would require two stitches to the chin.

Shaken up and not wanting to get wet, I stayed in the car, and soon, traffic was backing up on the road with people inching by the crash. Eventually, Jimmy emerged from the line of cars in their little Chevy Sonic, wondering what the backup was all about. Spotting me, Jimmy stopped, walked over to my car, and said in that calm, patient way: "Alright, Dick. Let's get you home."

I'd be fibbing if I told you I took this final defeat lying down. I blamed the truck, I blamed the rain, I'm sure I tried to find a way to blame the optometrist. I even vowed to go back down to the DMV, clear up the technicality, and claim my renewed and rightfully earned license.

Fortunately, age held the trump card: my eyes, by then, were officially shot. And there was no worming around that.

Back in the 1960s, after my first Jaguar's run-in with my first wall, the police said that I owed my survival to my seat belt; I was among the very few Americans at the time who wore one. So, I went out and told my whole story for a PSA advocating for seat belt usage.

In lieu of doing another PSA on "accepting that your driving days are done," I hope my story here will suffice. But it wouldn't be complete without a happy ending. Here, then are The Top Ten Things I Tolerate (and You Might Love!) About Being a Passenger:

10. I'm not worried about bumping other cars.
9. I can take my shoes off.
8. I can nap.
7. I can say "Wasn't that our turn?"
6. I get to hold the snacks.
5. I can look out the window all I want.
4. I can gaze at Arlene all I want.

3. I can make Arlene laugh by constantly mispronouncing signs. For instance, Chipotle, which I rhyme with *waddle*. "Chipoddel."
2. I can put both arms and all my body into the sing-along.
1. I still have myself, fully intact.

READ WHILE YOU CAN

I was a voracious reader, all through my life.

Mark Twain, tales of King Arthur, Isaac Asimov, the Tarzan series, dime-store pulp, the Bible, philosophy, psychology, scripts I was considering and scripts I'd done, the newspaper, fan mail, grocery lists, the answers on *Jeopardy!*, the crossword, street signs, prescription bottles.

Now it's all a blur. Literally. I can't, as they used to say, read a lick.

Up until a few years ago, reading glasses worked just fine. Every few years, I'd notice certain letters doubling up, or the smaller fonts getting fuzzy, and I'd run out for a stronger prescription.

Eventually, there was no prescription strong enough, and I turned to a magnifying glass. One of those big rectangular ones you scan over the page with, back and forth, back and forth. It was slightly nauseating, but it did the trick.

Then, quite suddenly, no magnifying glass in the world could make words come clear. Welcome to advanced dry macular degeneration.

I cannot describe just how shocking and awful this development has felt. Sure, I'm frustrated about blurry vision overall, but at least with some squinting, I can make out people's faces, the TV, or the shapes of clouds.

The written word, meanwhile, might as well be totally invisible. I've got books stacked in the bedroom that I've made notes in over the years, and both the books and my notes are totally useless to me now! A whole world I used to love and live in is now just gone.

No one told me this would happen!

Everything else in my body is fine, except for hearing and short-term memory and some foot issues. Those things, I had expected, and I've had time to get used to them and figure out decent enough workarounds. Right now, with reading, I'm still just in total, paralyzed disbelief.

I guess I could do books on tape, but those are best for novels where you go start to finish. The books I want to read are books you skip around in and peruse. Like this book on human behavior I have that has helped me understand acting (there's probably no audio version of that anyway). Or this philosopher who has this idea we all have an inner "ally" that's guiding us through life. Or the new Buster Keaton biography, so I can finally figure out how he did that spinning house bit!

Good luck finding what you need in the audio version of any of those.

I ask Arlene to read some stuff to me, and she does. But if I asked her to read everything I want to read, she would be chained to me for life.

Plus, reading is a solitary thing for me, and if I had someone reading aloud to me, I'd get distracted and start giving them notes on their delivery.

I keep thinking this is temporary, that one day, I'll look at a book and all the words will be clear again. Sadly, this is one part of aging that probably can't be reversed. All I can do now is work my way toward accepting that. When I do, I'll take out all my old Tarzans, squint to admire their ravishing cover artwork, which I hope will trigger memories of the stories inside.

DO GET ALL JUDGY (WHEN YOU'RE WATCHING TV)

Since books are too blurry for me these days, I've become a bit more of a couch/bed potato than I used to be. I shouldn't say "potato" because a potato isn't known for talking. When I'm watching TV, I talk a lot. Especially with Arlene around as my audience. She says watching TV with me is the greatest show on earth.

Well, sometimes the show can get a little peppery, I will admit. In the uninhibited anonymity of home, once the armchair critic in me gets wound up, it's hard to wind it back down. Moment by moment, show by show, I'm in a froth of nitpicking disapproval.

And guess what? It feels great! And it's good for me.

Nobody can be Mr. Nice Guy all the time! We all need to let ourselves get judgy every now and then, and as far as defendants go, there's plenty of evidence to find TV "guilty" on all sorts of counts.

Before I give you a taste of what a day in my court looks like, a caveat. I realize that there are human beings behind what I'm pecking away at on-screen. So, I respectfully apologize in advance if any of my pecking hurts a little. Please know it's all in fun . . . and take solace in the fact that, when I really get going, my beak spares no one.

Between each of my little diatribes, imagine my big index finger gleefully poking the remote as if to kill it, which is my way of changing channels, in search of a fresh target.

Jeopardy! Who dresses Ken Jennings?! He never gets a dimple on his tie, which drives me nuts! And he's got the one button buttoned on the jacket, which I originated, but his tie is hanging out below it! Wrong. You don't want the tie hanging out below the button! Every night, I am on his back.

Poke.

Entertainment Tonight. Who is that? Her again? Why?!

Poke.

Wicked. Do not get me started on how musical movies these days just butcher good choreography. All the cutting, cutting, cutting, the camera swooping and weaving. Whose legs are those? Why are they dancing in that giant library wheel?

Fred Astaire would never allow this. No dancer should, really.

I know I've been hard on the directors of *Mary Poppins* and *Chitty Chitty Bang Bang*, but one thing they both did right was to hold a shot for a good long time and keep it wide, so the audience could really see the whole number unfolding.

Nowadays, directors seem to believe that editing and cinematography are even more important than choreography. No, those first two are things we do with machines. Choreography is what we do with our bodies. Which do you really think is more fun to watch?

Poke.

Talk Shows. The guest and the host have just met each other. Why are they pretending to be best friends?

Political Shows. Everyone is reading from a teleprompter. Even the "arguments" are all planned out. How is this useful to anyone?

The Dick Van Dyke Show. Hmmm. Well, that didn't land at all.

Ritchie's smirking again.

What's with all these ads? It's all cut up!

Stop mugging, Dick!

Take it down a notch, Dick!

Now, if I'd paused and lifted my chin a tiny bit higher, *that* would have been funny.

LEARN A NEW WAY TO FALL

The other day, Jimmy came to work looking a little sore. "A fall went bad in the Battle Royale," they explained, pulling up a video on their phone for me to watch, "but it could have been a lot worse."

With that introduction, I wasn't sure I wanted to watch, but I did.

Let me explain. When Jimmy isn't helping me and Arlene, they are an actor, stuntperson, wrestling teacher, and, yes, a WWE-style wrestler! As in wild costumes, performative yelling and chest-thumping, body slams and throwing each other into the ropes. One of Jimmy's wrestling characters is American Oni, whose personality Jimmy describes like this: "basically me, Jimmy, dialed up to eleven." The "oni" is a character from Japanese folklore, a big superstrong demon-ogre thing (Jimmy is half Japanese).

After their matches, they always come in to work and show me clips. From a performance perspective, the strutting around larger-than-life costumed character stuff is hilarious and right up my alley. But the athletics of it and the stunts, all the violent throwing around and jumping, that stuff always takes me by surprise. Even though it's all planned out, a lot of those moves are actually very dangerous!

On this particular day, I found myself watching last weekend's Battle Royale. This is where a bunch of wrestlers are in the ring together, trying to eliminate their opponents by hurling them over the top rope and out of the ring. Count me out!

Jimmy narrated the mishap as I watched. A pair of opponents hoisted American Oni up for the over-the-ropes elimination, a stunt they'd all done plenty of times before.

"There are techniques for slowing yourself down as you're going over the rope," Jimmy explained, "but they got a little reckless, so I couldn't do anything. Basically, I just went over the top rope and straight onto the concrete."

"Oh my God!" I gasped at the phone. Even on the tiny screen, you could see just what a plummet it was. It was horrifying. And almost impossible for me to believe that Jimmy was standing there, alive to tell the tale.

Turns out, Jimmy explained, they had a secret weapon: martial arts muscle memory. Specifically, a technique called yoko ukemi, or "side breakfall," that protects your head and body during a fall.

"What?!" I exclaimed. Suddenly, I was more than just a prurient spectator. Jimmy had a new technique for falling, one that the Master of Pratfalls had never heard of. And now I wanted a lesson. "Show me!" Not a blurry video lesson; I wanted a live demo.

Jimmy eagerly obliged, narrating every step as they moved. Pull in your chin, bring your arm across your chest, palms down, swing your leg under and roll onto your side, bringing your full arm down against the ground as you hit.

As Jimmy explained and demonstrated, I just shook my head in awe. This was so much more complicated than Buster Keaton's "tuck and roll." Practically speaking, now that my own challenges with balance are real, not performed, this was stuff I could really use!

In senior living communities, I hear they have whole weekend-long seminars in how to safely fall. Maybe they would hire me and Jimmy. I could warm up the crowd with some patter and clips of my old pratfalls, then American Oni could strut in and do the teaching.

CARPE CHITA

During my run on Broadway with *Bye Bye Birdie*, Carl Reiner saw the show and was impressed enough with my performance to offer me the starring role in his new sitcom, which would become *The Dick Van Dyke Show*.

Sixty years later, my Broadway costar Chita Rivera confessed to me just how much my departure from the show had hurt at the time. "You abandoned us," she said, only half joking. Then she went on: "I never said this to anybody, but when that happened to you, I kind of went"—and here, she dropped her mouth into a dejected frown—"Well, [Carl] didn't really think I was good enough to write me into the series."

It really hurt to hear this. Because, looking into her eyes, I knew Chita wasn't saying it out of professional jealousy.

We had such chemistry in *Bye Bye Birdie*, Chita and me. We were *making things vibrate*, and she wanted to keep that going. As excited as I was to have a TV series, I wanted to keep it going too! When I left New York, I also left a chapter with Chita—or two or three chapters!—unfinished.

The occasion for this conversation was the 2021 Kennedy Center Honors, where I was an award honoree at ninety-six. Chita, who was eighty-eight, had gotten one herself two decades earlier. So there we sat with our matching rainbow-ribboned medals around our necks, having one of the most rewarding chats of my lifetime.

We volleyed story after story of *Bye Bye Birdie*. How each of us had come to the show. How anxious she'd been about kissing me during one rehearsal when my wife was sitting in. How hard it was for me to keep in character with all her comedic surprises:

"At any moment, I thought I'd just start laughing. Like: Okay, this is it. I'm just gonna go!'"

"And I would go anywhere you went!" Chita replied, beaming.

We talked a lot about performance in general. The importance of being "ready" when a new opportunity comes our way. The beauty of stumbling onto magic through accidents and experiments in rehearsal. And an incredible lesson that she'd learned from starting out in chorus lines: you always must know where you are within the group of other dancers. "You have to breathe each other."

Then we got around to marveling over how long it is we've both stuck around in the profession.

"Time is a fascinating thing. I don't know what it is," Chita said. "I just feel that I'm going to be here forever and I'm sure you do too."

"I couldn't stop entertaining for anything!" I replied.

"I couldn't either!"

Out of this effortless reunion, we picked up on the thread of our "unfinished business" together and hatched a rough plan to do a show, a revue of singing and storytelling. "We could do an hour and a half, easy!" I declared. "It would be like falling off a log!"

I don't know for sure about Chita, but it really felt like the excitement was mutual.

At the time, we were in the thick of COVID, of course, so everything in theater was on hold. We never really got any further with our dream after that. But I guess I thought, like Chita had said, we'd be here forever. We had all the time in the world to make our show happen together.

Chita died in January 2024, so I guess we were wrong.

I'm still sad that we never did that show. But as far as "next chapters" go, that conversation was darn near perfect.

REMEMBER HONESTLY

In my last book ten years ago, when I told the story of getting my first bike as a kid, I fudged the truth on a key detail. I'm coming clean now not just to clear my conscience.

Here's what I said then: When I was ten, I spotted a forlorn old junker of a bike in a pawnshop and begged my father for the seven dollars to buy it. Times were tight and so was his salary, so he resisted at first, then finally plunked down the cash. Once I'd cleaned that bike up, it was my ticket to boyhood freedom and fun.

A sunny story, right? I brought it up in my last book to help show how I've always been a kid at heart and how the freedom to "play" is what gives me spirit and life.

That part is absolutely true.

But I was so intent on putting a smile on my life experiences that I nudged the little hint of darkness out of the story. Here's the truth:

My father never gave me that seven dollars for the bike. He never gave me a single dollar for it. I earned three dollars from cutting grass, then begged my father for a four-dollar *loan* to cover the rest, which he finally agreed to, but only if I swore to pay it back. And I did pay it back in full.

At the time, this hurt. Of course, I now understand that my father really didn't have any money to spare at all. He had a meager salary from his job as a traveling salesman. We lived in a house owned by my mother's father, and our food and necessities came from my mother's father's grocery store. Times were tight.

Do I wish he had been a better dad to me and a better husband to my mother? Sure. On Saturday, his one day off, he wasn't out playing catch with his sons or helping his wife with the housework. He was out playing golf.

But I guess I'm sad about that more than angry. I just don't think he had it in him.

The root of the problem, I think, was that my father didn't really like himself. He was halfway decent on the horn around the house, though he never learned to read music, much less went out and played in public. He blamed his job for somehow keeping him from his calling as a musician, but the fact is he never really tried.

When I found my own calling in entertainment and struggled and worked to make it a reality, my father was generally proud and supportive. But sometimes it felt strange.

In the early 1950s, I had just landed a plum seven-year contract at CBS, and my parents came in from Illinois for a visit. One night, we took the train in from Long Island to have dinner at Danny's Hideaway, a steakhouse near Grand Central where all the TV people hung out.

For some reason, my father took me by the arm and walked me over to the bar and introduced me to an actor named Victor Jory, whom neither of us knew. "This is my son, Dick Van Dyke. He's on CBS!"

I smiled dutifully and shook hands, but inside I was uncomfortable. I know it came from a place of pride, but it felt over the top and out of the blue. I can't at all figure out what that was about.

Just a few years after this dinner, once I'd truly proven myself with *The Dick Van Dyke Show*, my father told me over the phone, with great relief, how proud he was of me. It came with a barb, though. He confessed to me that he and my mother had always worried that I wouldn't "amount to anything."

By this time in life, I was used to these sorts of offhand jabs, so I tried not to let it get to me. And for the most part, I have kept my more complicated feelings about my father to myself.

Part of this was to protect my brother Jerry, who idolized our father for his whole life. I'd always been hesitant to puncture or complicate Jerry's rosier vision, so I kept my feelings quiet.

There's another reason, too. I truly am an optimist at heart, as the rest of this book—and my life's body of work—makes clear. At the same time, I've felt pressure to be an optimist *unfailingly*. Which has meant tucking away stuff like that four-dollar loan for my bike.

All of which is to say: Whatever sunny "spin" we put on our childhoods may not be good for us in the long run. I've made peace with my mixed feelings for my father. And as soon as I acknowledged the real story of the bike, the weight of it disappeared. And bam! I forgave my dad in an instant. And the love I have for him came flooding back in.

LIVE WITH REGRETS

When it came to being a father myself, I always had my own dad in the back of my mind as an example of what not to do. And I think I did a very good job bettering him in all departments.

I supported my family financially, and I was happy about it. I spent what little free time I had at home with my family. I gave my kids a life of adventure and joy, a spirit to live their lives to the fullest. I set an example of decency and kindness, and when I saw those qualities blossoming in them, I nurtured them.

At the same time, I did fail. In the darkest days of my drinking, I was moody and lost my temper on occasion and I know that unsettled them. Once I was sober, I was honest about my remorse.

My biggest regret, though, is this persistent feeling that I was distant. That I wasn't there enough.

I was on the road an awful lot, in some other state or country filming, working all the time. It was a big happy reunion when I came home, but every time, there was always something in their lives I had missed. Birthdays, a new boyfriend, passing a big test. Beyond that, I wasn't there to experience how they were growing and changing as people, day to day.

I wish I had been more a part of that, helping them through their minor crises, seeing in the moment what their life's challenges were teaching them.

We have stayed connected through life, and we share Margie in our memories and hearts. They understand and trust my love with Arlene.

And of course, they've all become adults and had kids and grandkids of their own, and those families have become their primary ones. And you better believe it that all four of my children have been much better parents than I was. They are all very present.

It softens my feeling of regret to know that. It makes me proud.

YOUR PURPOSE DOESN'T NEED TO BE GRAND

Some people lean into being more of an "observer" as they grow older, and I can see how that could bring joy and satisfaction. But it's not me. I'll always be a "doer." My question now is: do what?

I keep thinking there must be a reason why I'm still alive, there's something I'm supposed to do. Otherwise, I just can't explain it. I don't know what that "thing" is though yet.

Luckily, in this time of limbo, I have my past as a guide. For my whole life, I've found my greatest sense of "purpose" in entertaining, in bringing laughter and joy to my fellow human beings. So, I know that's the arena I should be working in now.

But I wonder if it might be deeper than just song and dance. Honestly, I would like to do something—a play, a live show, a movie—that shows people how to love and care for one another again. That's a message that, at this point in my life, I feel uniquely suited to deliver. And it's a message that needs to be heard.

There's also politics. For my whole life, from the Civil Rights Movement to Proposition 8 in the 2000s, I've fought for equality and justice, what I believe in most passionately.

For two elections in a row, I threw myself into campaigning across the country for Bernie Sanders, who inspired me like no other politician before. And now he's out on the road again, shining a spotlight on just how dire our current political situation is. Bernie's no spring chicken, either; if he can still holler the truth, so can I!

Now, there are limits to my doer personality. In my career, it's never been me getting a big project off the ground, but rather somebody bringing one to me, and that's when I give "doing" my all. On top of that, now I have very real physical limitations, so what I want to do doesn't always match up with what I can do.

I suppose I could fritter my days away waiting for my purpose to reveal itself. But I might die before that happens!

Maybe I should stop thinking of all this so grandly, like I have to find the perfect thing.

So, yes, consider this my call to the universe: Send Dick Van Dyke a great script!

But in the meantime, while waiting for the universe to call back, I've just put in another call—to Bernie's office. Sign me up, buddy! Whatever help you need in the greater Los Angeles area that comes with a comfortable chair and a bottle of water, I'm your guy.

YOU WILL NOT BE ALONE

In 1987, my first grandchild Jessica, thirteen years old, took four baby aspirin to soothe a fever caused by chicken pox. Soon after, she grew disoriented, started vomiting, and was rushed to the hospital. Her brain was swelling, her kidneys and liver were failing, and she went blind.

Within a week, Jessica was gone. The aspirin had triggered a rare and little-known disease called Reye's syndrome.

Our entire extended family, Jessica's friends, schoolmates, and teachers, all of us were just broken. Together and alone, we agonized over one question more than any other: Why? I, for one, never came up with a good answer. By that point in my life, religious faith and a belief in a higher power were kind of shaky. Still, my only solace came from hoping that Jessica's spirit might be living on in some form or another.

Also, here in our world, her voice was still with us. Jessica had been a bold and startlingly deep thinker, curious and alive to hard questions about life, and she poured that into writing, poetry specifically. After she passed away, her parents compiled her poems into a book and gave a copy to everyone who knew her. I remember reading it for the first time, marveling and weeping.

Jessica was at that mysterious and fraught in-between age, neither child nor adult, and she was really looking inside herself and trying to make sense of things. Many of her poems are about the fragile blur between dreaming and awake, between life and death.

NIGHTMARES

In the dark I lie,
Paralyzed;
The world around me is forgotten,
Gone.
The nightmare creeps up into my brain,
Stealing consciousness.
It slithers over me like an evil snake.
Forgotten are warm friends and family;
For when I am forsaken in my nightmares,
I am but one creature,
Departed from life,
Lying desperately, trying to fight my
Nightmares.

Reading that poem for the first time, I was struck by how alike it was to the awful struggle Jessica had gone through as she was dying. I even imagined, somehow, that she had sensed what was going to happen to her when she wrote it.

That thought has ebbed over these thirty years, but the poem itself only keeps hitting me harder. I read it today and she is describing exactly what I'm going through.

I can feel the end of my life so much closer. All day, I seem to be dozing off or inching awake. The space between "being here" and "being gone" is just as Jessica described: a fragile blur.

And sometimes, that blur is as terrifying for me as it was for her. In the middle of the night, when my sleep is deepest, I'm at my most naked and vulnerable, and darkness, sadness, and loss just flood into my dreams. I ache for Arlene and for my family, for the feeling of being safe and not alone.

If I'm lucky, a visitor shows up in my nightmares. No, it isn't Jessica. It's my daughter Stacy, who passed away in 2017. I am sorry I can't bring myself to talk too much about the experience of losing her. Eight years later, the pain is still too awful. Stacy was my first daughter and held a supremely special place in my heart. She was a born performer and a gorgeous singer. Arlene adored Stacy, too, and our whole family is so thankful to have part of her still alive with us in her incredible son Ryan.

For all the sadness and loss, the feeling Stacy brings me in my dreams is the exact opposite. She's there. Right with me. Soothing me somehow, in a way that feels like magic. Telling me that, whatever happens, it's going to be okay, her warmth filling up inside me where fear used to be. We have found each other again, and we are together.

When I'm awake, that feeling of Stacy is still with me, a force of love and comfort I can wear like a blanket.

I also have a feeling of Jessica, though, who had described being trapped alone in her dream of death. It's horrible to think of her or Stacy like that.

But I imagine that if I had Stacy help me as a comfort in my dreams, then both she and Jessica had someone or something helping them on their own journey after life. Wherever their spirits went, I believe they are safe and they aren't alone.

And hopefully, when my time comes, they'll let me in there with them too.

SAVE THE AFTERLIFE FOR AFTER LIFE

In my waking and alert hours, I don't sit around thinking about death all the time. And I can't say I fear it either.

My spirit, my soul, whatever part of me that may still be left after my body is gone, I think I'll probably be okay. If that's my version of faith at this point, I'll take it. And I'll just keep hanging on to it as long as I can.

From a more rational perspective, what happens after life is a total unknown, like so much of the world. And I'm okay with that too. A few years ago, scientists discovered a planet thirty-one billion light-years away that might be the closest thing to Earth we've got out there. If we're just discovering this now, about one little speck so far away, that leaves an entire universe of things that are still a complete mystery.

So why would I just blindly hold on to some thin, little idea of a heaven or an afterlife or whatever, that in the grand scheme of things, was hatched in just a millisecond of the history of the universe?

As I see it, there are much more *knowable* things that we can and should hold on to. Most importantly, our outstanding obligations here on Earth now. How can we love and nourish our fellow beings, human and nonhumans alike, to improve our collective life here together?

We can't punt that one to God or the afterlife. That's on us.

In other words, don't ask me about dying because I still have a lot of important living to do. We all do.

YOU CAN'T PROTECT YOUR SURVIVORS

As I was putting this book together, the actor Gene Hackman and his wife Betsy died, along with one of their dogs, in their home in New Mexico. I followed the news about it every day, which brought to life more awful information and more mystery about their deaths, and how perilously alone their life had been before that.

I thought a lot about Gene during those weeks. He and I had grown up together in Danville, Illinois. He was the younger cousin of Bob Hackman, one of my teenage pals and a member of the Burfords. We'd be telling our jokes and doing our pranks, going way over the top, and Gene would just be along for the ride, not saying much, just quietly observing us.

Every time I saw him in a movie, I thought the same thing about his performance. He had so much internal power that he made everyone around them look like they were acting.

It finally came out that Betsy had died of the rodent-borne disease hantavirus, and that Gene, who was suffering from Alzheimer's, had lived alone in the house with his wife's body for a week before his own death from heart disease.

It was agony thinking about Gene during that week. In shock and anguish, terrified and completely lost. Maybe not even knowing where Betsy was in the house or realizing that she had died. Or worse, knowing and forgetting and then finding her and remembering again. It's too much sadness to take.

How could I also not think about myself. I have Arlene, who is in good health, and we have Jimmy, who is always here or close by. We have good neighbors, too, right next door. So, I don't worry about being isolated or not being cared for.

It's just the precarity of the whole thing that hits me. Anything could happen and I'd be gone in a second. At some level, I know this, and I've made peace with it. I'm not afraid of dying.

But at the same time, I know that what comes next, after I'm gone, will be awful. I went through it when I lost my ex-wife Margie and my partner Michelle. I've thought about it happening to Arlene, and I wish more than anything I could save her from it.

FIND YOUR ARLENE

The other day, I had a damn kidney stone. I have a high tolerance for pain, but a kidney stone is in a category all its own.

Arlene drove me into LA for a CT scan and it totally wiped me out. Then yesterday, we had to go to urgent care to get my levels checked.

A kidney stone is not going to be what kills me, but it sure felt like it was trying.

But I'm not here to complain. I'm here to tell you about what happened, on the way to the CT scan. I was in the passenger seat, barely able to keep it together, and Arlene did her magic on her phone and voilà, we're listening to Ella Fitzgerald's version of "It's Only a Paper Moon." One of our favorites.

Singing in the car is our sweet spot. We can ham it up, we can belt, we can riff and go all kinds of places we'd never dare to go onstage. Singing in the car with Arlene is my definition of eternal happiness.

Except on this particular day, I had a kidney stone and was in agony.

Still, Arlene had a plan, and she is not one to be discouraged. She started singing along to Ella, and I managed some humming/mumbling too.

It's a honky tonk parade
Without your love

This got us to what Arlene knows is my favorite lyric:

It's a melody played in a penny arcade

And with that, I'm in! "Great lyric!"

Now Arlene's singing and I'm "ba-dum-dumming" right along with her.

The music did not remove the pain. But it did carry my mind away from it. Which was Arlene's plan all along.

It's like that with so many things in our relationship. I assume things just magically happen, but in fact, they happen because Arlene has been working very hard to make them happen.

Months before my ninetieth birthday at Disneyland, Arlene was planning and wrangling for the park to pull out all the stops. While I was gazing fondly from my sit-up machine across the gym at her on the treadmill, she wasn't just flushed and dewy from her workout. She was on her phone emailing with Bob Iger's office! The head of Disney!

And when that birthday rolled around, it was the biggest and best of my entire life.

So many old celebrities just kind of fade out and are forgotten. But Arlene has made it the exact opposite for me. Back when Vines were whatever Vines were, Arlene had me doing them. She got me on Twitter and Instagram and everything else, which has connected me with my fans in a way I never had been before. And just this year, she has dreamed up Vandy Camp, a regular local family event featuring performances from us and the Vantastix and a host of other talented entertainers, conversations with fans, and all kinds of other, colorful fun. It just keeps getting bigger and better! Financial proceeds have gone to Malibu's Community Fire Brigade and other local businesses struggling after the recent wildfires. Emotional proceeds have gone to me, nearly a hundred and feeling more loved and purposeful than ever.

Nowadays, public reactions to me are becoming so much more emotional. I'm entering this strange territory where people think I have some kind of spiritual powers. A macho repair guy came over to our house, spotted me out by the pool, bit his knuckles and wept to Arlene and Jimmy: "That guy's a goddamn Buddha!"

I was eating a sandwich!

It always surprises me to experience all this love. It is an indescribably beautiful feeling, don't get me wrong. But I can't help but wonder: Would I be such a "national treasure" if it weren't for Arlene, tirelessly tooting my horn?

One of the hardest things about getting old is losing memory. It feels like whole parts of you are just being snatched away. I can't tell you how many times this pain has struck me over the past few years. I'll have the beginning of an old story, or the vague impression of a person I once knew, but the full thing isn't there.

Then, to my great surprise, Arlene comes to the rescue. It turns out, all these years we've been married, she hasn't just been listening to me; she's been remembering and packing away everything I say! Her strong, young mind has become my external hard drive, or my filing cabinet or whatever storage metaphor you prefer.

Arlene knows my entire life, from childhood right up to now. Well over three-quarters of the memories in this book were foggy in my brain but crystal clear in hers. It was Arlene who remembered that "What'd it run you?" came from my great-grandmother, how my belt buckle got stuck together with Chita Rivera's onstage, all the scary details of that men's room clown-killer. Arlene doesn't just remember the big picture of my stories either; she remembers the details, the nuances and the context which otherwise would have faded away.

"How do you know all this?!" I'll gasp.

"Because you told me," she'll reply matter-of-factly.

Arlene doesn't just *tell* me what I've forgotten, either; she makes me work for it. She asks me leading questions to get my memory up and running, so I can then fill things in on my own. This is an amazing technique: it helps me hold on to a story once it's resurfaced, then opens up all kinds of other memories around it too. How did she know how to do that?!

She does this with so many other of my age-related struggles. She doesn't force me to do things. She just lets me know that they're possible. When I complain that I've forgotten the words to a song, she'll put the music out on my bedside table. When I'm thinking maybe I'll skip the gym that morning, she'll walk back and forth in front of the TV in her workout clothes until I change my mind.

Self-deprecation comes all too easily these days. "I never really knew how to dance," I'll say. "I can't remember anything anymore." This annoys Arlene to no end, and she'll go toe to toe on why I'm wrong, every time. "You move like nobody else in the world!" "You just told stories for two straight hours!"

There's no denying how fragile living feels at this age. My mind and body are giving out in more ways than I can count, so things are always going askew. It's so easy to feel lost and powerless. But then, there is always Arlene, a force of calm and reassurance, somehow making my life still feel clear and graceful.

When I tell Bootsy that her bark is blowing out my hearing aids, Arlene reminds me that Bootsy is a dog. When I spiral into a rant about global politics, Arlene will put on a silly hat to get me laughing.

When she hears something crash from the other room, she doesn't panic. She smiles.

When she hears me singing "Hellloooo" from the other room, she assumes I'm singing a song like I always do. When my singing becomes more urgent, and she comes in to discover that I've gotten myself stuck upside down on the inversion board, she patiently helps me out of it and jokes that we now have material for a new episode of *The New New New Dick Van Dyke Show*.

Out of all the rules in this book, all the strategies for reaching one hundred I could ever dream of, finding my Arlene is the most important, hands down.

And *being* Arlene is something we should all aspire to. Not that we'll ever get there, because Arlene is in a category all her own, but we sure can try. Whether you're married or not, whether you're a spouse, a parent, a child, a sibling, a fast friend, an out-of-touch friend, a neighbor or a caregiver, everyone deserves the purpose and joy Arlene has given me.

When I say I'm old, Arlene shows me all the ways I am young.

When I worry about death, she tells me I am life.

When darkness creeps in, she turns on the magic.

Now you try it. Be Arlene.

When darkness creeps in, turn on the magic.

About the Author

Dick Van Dyke is an American actor, singer, entertainer, comedian, and producer. His award-winning career has spanned seven decades in film, television, and stage. Van Dyke began his career as an entertainer on radio and television, in nightclubs, and on the Broadway stage. In 1961, he starred in the original production of *Bye Bye Birdie* alongside Chita Rivera, a role that earned him the Tony Award for Best Featured Actor in a Musical. Carl Reiner then cast him as Rob Petrie on the CBS television sitcom *The Dick Van Dyke Show (*1961–1966), which made him a household name. He went on to star in the motion picture musicals *Bye Bye Birdie* (1963), *Mary Poppins* (1964), and *Chitty Chitty Bang Bang* (1968), and in the comedy-drama *The Comic* (1969). He made guest appearances on television programs *Columbo* (1974) and *The Carol Burnett Show* (1977), and starred in *The New Dick Van Dyke Show* (1971–74), *Diagnosis: Murder* (1993–2001), and *Murder 101* (2006–08). Van Dyke has also made appearances in the motion pictures *Dick Tracy* (1990), *Curious George* (2006), *Night at the Museum* (2006), *Night at the Museum: Secret of the Tomb* (2014), and *Mary Poppins Returns* (2018).

Van Dyke is the recipient of five Primetime Emmys, a Golden Globe, a Tony, and a Grammy Award, and was inducted into the Television Hall of Fame in 1995. He received the Screen Actors Guild's highest honor, the SAG Life Achievement Award, in 2013. He has a star on the Hollywood Walk of Fame at 7021 Hollywood Boulevard and has also been recognized as a Disney Legend. In 2021, Van Dyke was honored with the Kennedy Center Honors.